teach®
yourself

breastfeeding

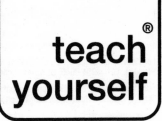

breastfeeding
pauline lim

Launched in 1938, the **teach yourself** series grew rapidly in response to the world's wartime needs. Loved and trusted by over 50 million readers, the series has continued to respond to society's changing interests and passions and now, 70 years on, includes over 500 titles, from Arabic and Beekeeping to Yoga and Zulu. What would you like to learn?

be where you want to be with **teach yourself**

For UK order enquiries: please contact Bookpoint Ltd, 130 Milton Park, Abingdon, Oxon OX14 4SB. Telephone: +44 (0) 1235 827720. Fax: +44 (0) 1235 400454. Lines are open 09.00–17.00, Monday to Saturday, with a 24-hour message answering service. Details about our titles and how to order are available at www.teachyourself.co.uk

For USA order enquiries: please contact McGraw-Hill Customer Services, PO Box 545, Blacklick, OH 43004-0545, USA. Telephone: 1-800-722-4726. Fax: 1-614-755-5645.

For Canada order enquiries: please contact McGraw-Hill Ryerson Ltd, 300 Water St, Whitby, Ontario L1N 9B6, Canada. Telephone: 905 430 5000. Fax: 905 430 5020.

Long renowned as the authoritative source for self-guided learning – with more than 50 million copies sold worldwide – the **teach yourself** series includes over 500 titles in the fields of languages, crafts, hobbies, business, computing and education.

British Library Cataloguing in Publication Data: a catalogue record for this title is available from the British Library.

Library of Congress Catalog Card Number: on file.

First published in UK 2008 by Hodder Education, part of Hachette UK, 338 Euston Road, London, NW1 3BH.

First published in US 2008 by The McGraw-Hill Companies, Inc.

This edition published 2008.

The **teach yourself** name is a registered trade mark of Hodder Headline.

Typeset by Transet Limited, Coventry, England.
Printed in Great Britain for Hodder Education, an Hachette UK Company, 338 Euston Road, London NW1 3BH, by CPI Cox & Wyman, Reading, Berkshire RG1 8EX.

The publisher has used its best endeavours to ensure that the URLs for external websites referred to in this book are correct and active at the time of going to press. However, the publisher and the author have no responsibility for the websites and can make no guarantee that a site will remain live or that the content will remain relevant, decent or appropriate.

Hachette UK's policy is to use papers that are natural, renewable and recyclable products and made from wood grown in sustainable forests. The logging and manufacturing processes are expected to conform to the environmental regulations of the country of origin.

Impression number   10 9 8 7 6 5 4 3 2 1
Year   2012 2011 2010 2009 2008

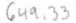

contents

acknowledgements

Thanks must go

to Victoria Roddam, for her support and patience in the development of this book

to Vicky and Jo for their helpful suggestions

also to my good friend, Babs, who would happily read endless chapters and give me her thoughts

to my family, husband Steve, Mat and Natasha, for listening to my concerns.

Finally, thank you to all the mums and babies for whom it has been my privilege to share their special times and I hope this book will be helpful to many others in their quest to breastfeed their babies.

Happy Breastfeeding!

introduction

As a midwife for over 20 years, and as an experienced breastfeeding mother myself, I firmly believe that breastfeeding is the best thing you can do for your baby.

The intention of this book is to enable you to make an informed decision about breastfeeding and to give you the support you need in making that decision, while also being realistic. I am wholly pro-breastfeeding and believe that if a mother really wants to breastfeed there is an extremely high likelihood that she will be successful. However, if you are not fully convinced then I hope this book will go some way to helping you make that decision.

Breastfeeding provides many health benefits for both you and your baby that cannot be gained from any other feeding method. The ideal is for you to be able to breastfeed your baby for the first six months of life. Many women start breastfeeding with high hopes but, unfortunately, within six weeks over 60% of them have given up. A huge part of being able to continue to breastfeed is overcoming any concerns or problems you encounter. That is where this book comes in.

In order to make a decision you need to have thought through the reasons why you wish to breastfeed. You need to have decided, for yourself, that breastfeeding is what you want, not just something your midwife or your partner/mum wants and expects you to do. Only then will you understand that you need to be prepared to work at it.

You will find information about your breasts and the changes to expect within them in Chapter 01, and details about why breast milk and breastfeeding are so good for you and your baby in Chapter 02.

Chapter 03 will help get you started, from right after your delivery. Chapter 04 concentrates on the issues of breastfeeding while you are in hospital and Chapter 05 offers advice to help you cope once you get home.

Many mothers will have a wonderful, problem-free breastfeeding experience, but for those who don't, Chapters 06 and 07 look at the problems you and your baby may encounter.

If you have questions about the need to supplement your breastfeeding, or how and when to introduce solid food, Chapters 08 and 10 may be useful.

In order to help you breastfeed, you will need to draw on the support of your partner, friends and family. Chapter 09 may be a useful read for you and those around you.

Chapter 11 discusses what improvements are being made within maternity care to help improve breastfeeding support and, ultimately, breastfeeding rates. It includes a section about breastfeeding in public. It is quite normal to see naked women displayed within our daily newspaper, but breastfeeding is still not really accepted within our society. It is hoped that some of the suggestions within this chapter will help to liberate you as a breastfeeding mother.

When writing this book I realized that many readers may not read it from cover to cover, but may refer to the parts that seem relevant to them at specific times. So, for this reason, there will be some repetition of key points rather than too much cross-referencing.

Throughout the book, for ease of use, I have used 'he/him' to refer to your baby and, rather than listing husband/partner/other half, I have maintained the term 'partner' as this is relevant to all.

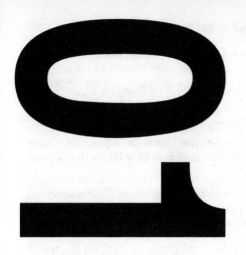

01

about your breasts

In this chapter you will learn:
- what your breasts look like
- how your breasts will change during your pregnancy
- about colostrum
- how your hormones affect your milk supply.

Development of the breast

You may not have looked closely at your breasts recently, perhaps not since you were a teenager when your body and breasts first started to develop. But, of course, you will have noticed that your breasts have changed during your pregnancy. They have probably changed in size or have felt quite tender, especially in the early weeks of your pregnancy. To help you feel prepared for the changes you will experience, let's look more closely at this part of your body, which is key to successful breastfeeding.

Your breasts start to develop during puberty but really only complete their development during pregnancy. This happens as a result of the hormones circulating in your body at that time. During this time your breasts will increase in size and you will see the nipple area darken. You may notice your breasts feeling larger, more tense and tingling, even during the first couple of months. For some women who have been pregnant previously, this may be one of the first signs they recognize as signalling that they are pregnant.

Most women will experience a gradual increase in the size of their breasts during pregnancy, although occasionally some women may experience a sudden spurt in the growth of their breasts. The average weight of an adult breast is between 150 and 200 grams (about six ounces) but this doubles during lactation to around 400 to 500 grams (up to about a pound). So you will need to ensure that your breasts are well supported during your pregnancy in order that you feel comfortable. You will need to be refitted for your bra during your pregnancy, possibly several times, early in your pregnancy and then a little later. If you are intending to breastfeed you will need to be fitted for a 'nursing' bra towards the end of your pregnancy, although you may find you can take a more accurate measurement after the first couple of weeks when your milk has 'come in'. (This phrase is used to describe the onset of mature breast milk production, as opposed to colostrum – see below. This usually takes 3–4 days and you will notice your breasts feel firmer and more full.)

Size and shape

Q. My breasts are normally small. Will I still be able to feed my baby?

Don't worry if your breasts are normally small, they will increase in size during pregnancy as the hormones increase the number of structures (ducts and alveoli – see page 4) within the breast. Everyone's breasts will be a different size – this has no bearing on how well you may be able to breastfeed. Your ability to breastfeed does not depend on the size of your breasts. It is very rare that your breasts will not be suitable for breastfeeding, unless you have had any breast surgery.

Q. My breasts are different sizes. Does it matter?

Most women have different sized breasts, the left often being larger than the right – again, this is quite normal and nothing to worry about.

Q. Will breastfeeding affect the size and shape of my breasts?

In most cases, the answer will be 'yes'! But so will pregnancy itself. Some women will have a much fuller breast size after breastfeeding, while others will find that their breasts shrink after breastfeeding. It can be difficult to predict what will happen for each individual. After pregnancy, your breasts will tend to hang lower anyway; this is often due to the amount of stretch and strain put on the ligaments of your breast as they grow. This is one reason why it is important to wear a supportive bra throughout pregnancy.

The nipples

Q. My nipples don't seem to be the right shape and size – they're flat. Will this affect my chances of breastfeeding?

Don't worry about the shape and size of your nipples. Most women's nipples protrude, but some are flat or inverted. You can determine whether your nipples are inverted by looking to see if they retract into the breast tissue, rather than sticking out, when you are cold or if you try to press your breast tissue around the darkened breast tissue (areola) with your fingers. See the diagram on page 110. You may just have one inverted nipple and one protruding nipple.

In the past, women with inverted nipples were sometimes advised to perform a number of exercises to 'prepare' the nipples for breastfeeding. However, this is not necessary – recent research that looked at nipple preparation for inverted nipples found it was of no value, whether using nipple 'shells' or 'stretching exercises'. An inverted nipple shouldn't affect breastfeeding as your baby does not feed just from the nipple but from the whole of the areola. However, it is important to make sure you have help from your midwife with the first few feeds to ensure that your baby is latching on correctly.

Inside your breasts

Inside your breast are special 'sacs' called alveoli, lined with special cells which are responsible for milk production. Milk is made up of lots of small droplets, which all join together, flow along the ducts and exit from about four to nine openings in the nipple. The milk ducts and cells inside your breast are separated by fibres, which help to create separate sections, or lobes. These help prevent any infection spreading throughout the breast, as it would be contained just to that section (or lobe). However, these fibres do not support your breast in any way, so it is important for you to wear a good supporting bra. Around the alveoli cells are more cells, which contract in response to a hormone (oxytocin) released by your body. It is this contraction – known as 'letdown' – that causes the milk to be forced out. Once you have been breastfeeding for a while you may notice this contraction as a tingling sensation within the breast.

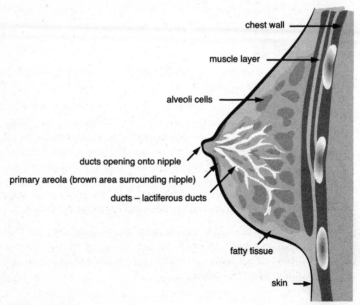

chest wall

muscle layer

alveoli cells

ducts opening onto nipple

primary areola (brown area surrounding nipple)

ducts – lactiferous ducts

fatty tissue

skin

figure 1.1 inside your breast

Top tip

Try not to compare your baby with any other, whether breast- or bottle-feeding, but adopt a 'baby-led' approach. Be ready to feed your baby when he is ready and let him come off the breast when he wants. This approach is sometimes called 'demand feeding'.

Hormones affecting your milk supply

Throughout your pregnancy your body is affected by a number of hormones.

Oestrogen and progesterone

- **Oestrogen** helps the ducts in your breast to develop.
- **Progesterone** helps to develop the glandular tissue in the breast. Once you have delivered the 'afterbirth' (placenta), levels of progesterone fall dramatically. If there are any pieces of placenta left inside your womb/uterus they may cause progesterone to continue to inhibit your lactation. This will usually by noticed by the midwife following delivery.

Prolactin

Prolactin is produced by the anterior pituitary gland (the front – anterior – section of the pea-sized pituitary gland, found at the base of the brain) throughout pregnancy, increasing in amounts until it reaches a maximum as you reach 'term'. This is the milk-producing hormone. Its effects are limited by the other hormones present during pregnancy, particularly progesterone and possibly oestrogen, which means that full milk production cannot happen until after delivery. Once you have delivered your baby there is a reduction in the level of these hormones (which the placenta has been producing to help your baby grow), so then prolactin can start to work properly.

Q. Is it necessary to breastfeed at night?

It is very important to breastfeed at night. Prolactin initiates and maintains your milk production. It is secreted at a stable level but extra bursts of prolactin are also released when you are breastfeeding. This stimulates the special cells in your breast to produce milk. These bursts of prolactin release are actually greater at night and during sleep, so it is very important to breastfeed your baby during the night in the early weeks as this will increase the amount of breast milk you produce.

Q. Why is it important to breastfeed frequently?

Prolactin levels are responsible for producing the next feed, so the more the baby suckles the more milk the breasts will make.

Prolactin levels almost double while you are breastfeeding and the increased production lasts for up to 45 minutes from the start of the feed. The levels then gradually decrease over the next couple of hours, by which time your breastfed baby will usually be ready to feed again.

Prolactin levels also rise with the frequency of feeds. If you can feed more than eight times in a 24-hour period it will help your breastfeeding, as the levels of prolactin will not drop too much in between feeds. The more frequently you breastfeed the more milk will be produced. So if possible, feed your baby at least two-hourly in the first few days.

Having said this, usually if your baby is born healthy and at term, he will regulate his own feeding pattern ('baby-led' feeding) which will usually be at around the two-hourly frequency. Babies are able to regulate their own calorie or fat intake, which means that they will take in the amount they need over time; this may not be the same every day but may actually balance out over a couple of days. So your body will respond and supply sufficient milk, provided that nothing interferes with this process.

Q. Will I have enough milk if I have twins?

The level of prolactin increases each time you breastfeed and this means more milk is produced. So if you have more than one baby there will be even greater stimulation of prolactin and so your milk supply will increase. So, if you are breastfeeding twins you will have sufficient breast milk.

Rarely is a mother unable to supply sufficient milk to feed her baby, but you should ensure you breastfeed your baby as often as he needs and give him only breast milk, which will allow your body to respond to his needs fully.

Important facts about prolactin

- Levels tend to be higher during the night (when you have been sleeping) than during the day.
- Prolactin levels remain raised for as long as you breastfeed (even for years), although the level does decline slowly from the initial high level.
- Levels rise with suckling, so the more frequently the baby feeds, the higher the levels of prolactin will be.
- More than eight feeds in 24 hours helps to maintain the levels of prolactin and ensure good milk production.
- Prolactin levels are increased when more than one baby is being breastfed.
- High prolactin levels delay ovulation, although it is not possible to predict when this wears off.
- Smoking cigarettes can reduce the level of prolactin and may reduce the amount of milk produced. Try to give up if you haven't already, or at least try to cut down.

Oxytocin

Oxytocin is a hormone produced by the posterior (towards the back of the head) part of the pituitary gland and is responsible for milk ejection or 'letdown'. Oxytocin is released when your baby cries, as your body prepares to feed your baby. It is closely linked to bonding and has been called 'the cuddle hormone'.

Q. Why do my breasts leak milk when my baby cries?

Oxytocin is released as your baby cries, so you may find your milk leaking when you can hear him crying or stirring. If you have your baby close to your bed at night ('rooming-in'), his cry or murmuring will help to signal to your body that he is ready to feed.

Oxytocin is released in waves and these seem to follow your baby's suckling pattern. Your breastfeeding baby will suckle for short bursts and then pause before suckling again; this matches the waves of oxytocin.

Q. What can stop my 'letdown'?

Oxytocin can trigger your milk letdown, but if you are tense, worried or anxious this can inhibit oxytocin and so prevent milk ejection. If this response is inhibited it is likely that part of the feed may not be letdown, so your baby will not get as much milk and will not be satisfied. You need to feel confident that you are able to feed your baby – your midwife will help you to develop the skills you need to avoid inhibiting the production of oxytocin.

You can encourage the oxytocin response by looking at and touching your baby. Having your baby or a photograph of him close to you can also have a positive effect on your letdown. If you have to be separated from your baby for any time, for example if he needs to be in a Special Care or Neonatal Unit, then keep a photograph by you or try to visit as often as you can, and this can help if you then try to express your milk.

Oxytocin produced during feeding will also affect the uterus in the form of 'mini-contractions'. You may feel these after-pains while you are feeding – remember, they are helping you to regain your shape. Your breasts may also tingle while you are feeding as the oxytocin stimulates the milk letdown reflex.

How do you know if oxytocin is being released?

- Your breasts may tingle before or during a feed.
- Milk may leak when your baby cries, or from one breast while you are feeding from the other.
- You may notice a fine 'jet' of milk flowing from your breast if your baby comes off the breast during a feed.
- You may feel abdominal or uterine cramps while feeding and for up to 20 minutes afterwards.
- You may notice increased vaginal blood loss during feeds in the first week, as your uterus contracts during breastfeeding.
- Your baby's suckling pattern will change from short sucks to slow deep suckling, and swallowing will be heard.
- You may feel thirsty while feeding.

Q. Why don't I need to breastfeed from both sides at each feed?

Apart from the hormones that are involved in the control of breast milk production, there is also control from within the breast itself. Breast milk contains a particular protein substance which will stop milk production when necessary. So it is possible that milk production will stop or reduce in one breast while continuing in the other breast. This may depend upon whether the baby feeds from each breast equally at each feed. Whether or not to feed at both breasts will depend on you and your baby – this will be discussed later.

Sometimes, if your breasts become very engorged this can stop the cells surrounding the milk sac from contracting. In this case it may be useful for you initially to try to hand-express a little of your breast milk.

Feeding your baby – suckling

I use the word *suckling* rather than *sucking* to describe how your baby obtains your breast milk. This is because when we think of sucking, we tend to think of an action similar to sucking using a straw. Suckling is a very different action. Your baby gets his milk feed by using his tongue, together with his jaw movements, to squeeze the breast tissues against the top of his mouth, and so pushes the milk along the milk ducts. So he actually has to do a lot of work to get the milk from your breast, whereas if he is fed from a bottle all he has to do is swallow as the milk drips into his mouth from the teat.

There is also, of course, the letdown reflex, which occurs as the milk sacs contract in response to the hormone oxytocin. When your baby is well positioned and latched on correctly, your nipple will actually extend far into his mouth. In fact, the opening of your nipple ducts will be right at the back of his mouth. This allows the whole of your baby's tongue to be involved in moving upwards in the mouth and so stroking along the underside of your breast tissue, while squeezing the breast against the upper part (soft palate) of his mouth. This compression movement happens rhythmically and so pushes the milk along the milk ducts and then into the back of the mouth, where your baby can then swallow it.

When your baby first comes off the breast, you should notice that the shape of your nipple and areola have changed. They will have become elongated, forming a teat shape which lies in the well of the tongue, which forms a scoop shape. Your baby's jaws should fit firmly around the areola tissue so there is no movement of the breast at all during suckling. This will ensure there is no friction against the nipple which could make you sore. If you do find you are becoming sore or feeling any pain it will usually mean your baby is not attached properly, so you need to check his feeding position.

Top tip

If you feel any pain, this is a warning sign that your baby is not positioned correctly and this may cause damage to your nipple. Remove your baby from the breast (by breaking the seal) and reposition him.

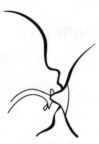

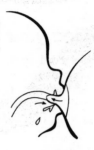

figure 1.2 attachment of baby at the breast (Royal College of Midwives, *Successful Breastfeeding*)

a) Shows the baby attaching to the breast.

b) Shows jaws clamping around the areola and cheeks then contracting. The tongue moves forward to scoop under the nipple/areola area.

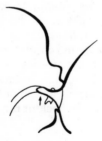

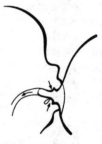

c) Shows the tongue moving upwards to compress the 'teat', which is formed by the nipple and areola tissue, against the roof of the mouth.

d) Shows the tongue compressing and then releasing the 'teat' – milk is actively removed and, as the teat is positioned towards the back of the palate, this is then swallowed.

02

benefits of breastfeeding

In this chapter you will learn:
- what your breast milk contains
- the benefits of breastfeeding for your baby
- the benefits of breastfeeding for you.

There are a number of benefits as a result of breastfeeding – this chapter will discuss what these are for you and your baby.

Nutritional benefits

The nature of the milk

Breast milk is the ideal milk for your baby. Its composition is perfect – it is custom made for your baby, whatever age he is and whenever he arrives. If your baby is born early (prematurely) your breast milk will still be ideally suited to meet his nutritional needs.

Your breast milk will change over time, ensuring it provides your baby with the correct nutrients he needs at that time, i.e. it is biologically specific for your child.

It helps keep allergies at bay – your baby will not be allergic to your breast milk, although if you have eaten something your baby is sensitive to this could be passed on in your milk.

Breast milk is completely nutritionally balanced. It is easily digested by a newborn baby due to the types of protein it contains.

What does breast milk contain?

Protein

Breast milk primarily consists of two types of protein, whey and casein. In the early days after birth, breast milk will contain mostly whey. Whey is much easier for the newborn baby to digest as it forms soft flaky curds.

Whey also contains other substances that help your baby's immune defence:

- Lactoferrin binds with iron in your baby and so prevents any bacteria from growing (which need iron).
- Lysozymes help kill bacteria and viruses.
- Immunoglobulins are antibodies that help pass on to your baby any immunity you have built up.

None of these anti-infective properties can be found in any formula milk.

In mature milk the whey–casein ratio is higher, although still in favour of whey. Only in later stages of lactation do these levels actually become equal.

Casein is the protein that satisfies the 'hungrier' baby, so as your baby grows this type of protein becomes more appropriate. In the early days it is difficult for your baby to digest casein as it forms tougher curds, which take longer to digest and uses more energy to do so.

Formula (artificial) milk contains more casein, which is why babies last longer between feeds as they feel full for longer. In the newborn baby this means digestion is less complete.

Carbohydrate

Lactose is the main carbohydrate, or sugar, found in breast milk.

- There is a high level of lactose in breast milk as it supplies the energy needed for baby's rapidly developing brain.
- Lactose makes breast milk taste sweeter.
- Lactose helps calcium to be absorbed. This is necessary for the development of strong teeth and bones. Although there are only small amounts of calcium in breast milk it is absorbed better than calcium from other sources.

Some of the other sugars found in breast milk promote the development of another substance known as *Lactobacillus bifidus*, which makes the gut more acid, thus helping to stop harmful bacteria from growing.

Fat

Fat is a major source of energy. The amount of fat in the breast milk varies depending on the gestation of your baby (i.e. at what stage of pregnancy you delivered and whether he was premature or term). The amount then changes to make sure your baby receives the correct balance at whatever age he is, varying according to the time of day he is fed (more late afternoon/early evening); and the duration of the both the feed (more during a longer feed) and the length of time you have been breastfeeding your baby for (i.e. from when you started to whatever age he is when you stop). It can also be affected by your diet (more if you have a healthy, balanced diet), how many babies you have had (tends to reduce the more children you have) and the time of year (more during winter).

Your breast milk also contains an enzyme that helps your baby to digest this fat.

Q. Why does my milk look watery at the start of a feed?

The fat content of the milk gradually increases during a feed, so that the milk at the beginning of the feed (known as 'fore milk') contains much less fat than milk produced towards the end of the feed ('hind milk'). The appearance of your milk may reflect this difference; the fore milk often appears watery or bluish in colour while the hind milk seems creamier and more dense.

If your baby feeds for short periods he may receive a larger volume of less calorific milk, which may be just what he needs at that time, for example in hot weather as a 'thirst-quencher'. However, if he always takes short feeds then he may not be getting all the fat-rich hind milk containing more calories.

There are a number of essential fatty acids, some of which are only found in breast milk while the concentration of others varies in cows' milk. These are all necessary for the baby's growing brain and eyes, as well as healthy blood vessels. There has been some suggestion that babies fed on milks lacking these may have poorer mental development and eyesight. These essential fatty acids have a higher proportion of unsaturated and long-chain fatty acids, which are absorbed better than saturated fats and account for the improved brain and sensory development.

The type of fat contained in your diet does influence the composition of fatty acids in breast milk, but does not affect the total amount of fat in the milk overall.

Cholesterol
Cholesterol helps with the development of the nervous system and is found in higher levels in breast milk than in formula milk, although this does change as your baby gets older.

Q. I thought cholesterol was 'bad' for you?

That's right, normally higher levels of cholesterol are not encouraged, but the reverse is true in the breastfed infant. This is because your baby's body adapts and can learn to break down cholesterol more effectively. This helps with long-term cardiovascular health.

Vitamins
The amounts of the different vitamins in breast milk will vary between individuals, depending partly upon diet.

Some vitamins are fat-soluble (A, D, E and K), and these can be taken from your body's stores. The higher the fat content of your breast milk, the higher the proportions of fat-soluble vitamins, so it is important that your baby feeds for as long as he wishes in order to ensure that he gets the fat-rich hind milk.

- **Vitamin A** is responsible for the development of your baby's eyes. There are more than adequate amounts in your breast milk if you are eating well yourself.
- **Vitamin D** production requires sunlight, so if your baby is not exposed to sunlight he may be deficient in this vitamin. Levels of vitamin D in breast milk are a little low, but it is very rare for breastfed infants to develop rickets as a result.
- **Vitamin K** is essential to help blood to clot. The levels of vitamin K are higher in colostrum and hind milk, so it is very important to make sure your baby takes this. It will eventually be produced naturally in the gut of the baby, but initially the gut is sterile, so it can take up to six weeks to reach adequate production.
- **Vitamin B complex** and high levels of **vitamin C** are found in breast milk. Vitamin C helps iron to be absorbed, whilst vitamin B is involved in a variety of body processes, including development of the nervous system and blood cells.

Iron

Iron helps in the formation of blood. Your baby will store iron in his body during the latter weeks of your pregnancy. Although there are only small amounts of iron in breast milk, it is absorbed more efficiently because it is helped by the vitamin C also present in the breastmilk.

Iron helps to prevent anaemia, but your baby does not need excess iron. Too much iron can stop lactoferrin from being effective as it cannot be 'mopped up' and so can be used by the harmful bacteria in the gut to grow and reproduce.

Benefits of breastfeeding for your baby

Your breast milk is ideally balanced for your baby. It changes during each feed and throughout the time of your lactation overall. If you breastfeed exclusively this will ensure that your baby receives the correct amount of nutrients and enjoys the other benefits of breast milk.

Q. Will giving my baby formula milk have any effect?

Giving a bottle can change the state of your baby's gut, which may lead to him becoming sensitized. This can mean he is more likely to develop allergies later on.

Your baby has only limited ability to digest foods when he is newborn. During the first three months of life your baby's ability to digest foodstuffs does not change very much, but after this his organs will have matured sufficiently to be able to cope with most other foods.

The effect of breastfeeding on jaw development

In order to breastfeed properly your baby has to work his jaw and surrounding muscles. This will help him develop strong jaw muscles and, because of this, support his speech development.

The feeding action also helps to keep the tube between the back of the throat and the ear (the Eustachian tube) open, which can reduce his chances of *otitis media* (middle-ear infections). The breastfeeding action will also increase your baby's protection against dental decay and possible overcrowding of the teeth.

Breast milk as an anti-allergenic

Because your breast milk contains anti-allergenic agents your baby is less likely to develop an allergy. His general health will be better too; breastfed babies have fewer infections so are less likely to suffer gastric, respiratory and urinary infections during infancy.

Breast milk and obesity

If you are worried about the rising levels of obesity and childhood diabetes, breastfeeding can help to decrease your baby's likelihood of developing either. Although breastfed babies often gain weight more rapidly during the first two months, they generally weigh less (on average) at one year than a formula-fed infant, even once started on solids. This is because the breastfed baby controls the amount of milk he takes; because he stops when he feels full his stomach will not become overstretched. Also, because your baby has to work hard to get the milk he will stop when he has had enough as it will be quite tiring for him.

If a baby's stomach is overstretched regularly, the baby will become accustomed to this 'full' feeling. Then your baby will expect this feeling each time he feeds and so this can become the habit for life, leading to overfeeding and then overeating.

Breast milk and neural development

Breastfed babies have improved brain, central nervous system and sensory development. Breastfed babies will tend to have higher IQs at ages 11 and 16 years.

Benefits of breastfeeding for your baby

- He receives the exact breast milk composition he requires at whatever age he is.
- It enhances jaw and tongue development.
- It improves speech development.
- It can protect against *otitis media* and many respiratory, urinary and gastric infections.
- It can reduce the incidence of dental decay and overcrowding of teeth.
- Breastfed infants have lower blood pressure during childhood and early teenage years.
- There is less likelihood of developing severe allergies.
- There is less likelihood of sudden infant death in breastfed infants.
- The incidence of obesity and diabetes is reduced.
- Brain, sensory and neurological developments are improved.

If you would like further information about the benefits of breastfeeding, look at the National Childbirth Trust or La Leche League websites or The Royal College of Midwives book – *Successful Breastfeeding*. Contact details and further information will be found in the 'Taking it further' section at the back of this book.

Benefits for mother

We've looked at why breastfeeding might be good for your baby, but does it offer any benefits for you?

Convenience

An obvious advantage for you is the convenience of breastfeeding – there is no need to prepare bottles of formula milk. Breast milk is always available, at the correct temperature. You won't need to worry about making up a feed on time or have to get up in the middle of the night to prepare a feed.

You will need to take frequent rest periods, although you may not always appreciate these. The hormones released during breastfeeding are also very calming, so you will feel relaxed during and shortly after a feed. So if you breastfeed during the night you will be more able to relax and go back to sleep.

Energy consumption (and potential weight loss)

Breastfeeding does use up a lot of energy and, therefore, calories. However, don't be tempted to overeat – simply eat and drink a normal healthy balanced diet to satisfy your own hunger and thirst; although I would recommend that you have a drink beside you while you are feeding your baby. You can lose weight more rapidly if you breastfeed in the first three to six months post-delivery.

Breastfeeding will also help you regain your pre-pregnancy weight and shape because the hormone oxytocin will cause the cells in the wall of your uterus (womb) to contract. Due to these contractions you will find that you tend to have heavier vaginal blood loss, which will also mean that this blood loss ends sooner; this can help reduce your risk of becoming anaemic.

Financial benefits

There will be obvious financial benefits as there is no need to buy any formula milk, bottles, brushes, etc. There will be no wasted 'half-used' bottles.

There are also some less immediate and less obvious financial benefits, given the numerous health benefits to both you and your baby. Your child is likely to have fewer frequent illnesses and fewer allergies, which will lead to a reduction in healthcare costs – not just for the individual but for society as a whole.

Other possible benefits

- Breastfeeding for at least six months may reduce the risk of some ovarian and pre-menopausal breast cancers.
- Breastfeeding mothers are less likely to develop osteoporosis and there is a lower incidence of hip fractures in women over 65 years of age who breastfed.
- Breastfeeding is one factor that can help to reduce post-partum depression.

- Diabetic mothers may need less medication or insulin while breastfeeding. If you have had gestational diabetes during your pregnancy you may find feeding (and the amount of calories this will use) can help you reach a more optimal weight and therefore reduce the risk of developing diabetes.
- Breastfed babies automatically receive a variety of flavours in your breast milk, which obviously depends on your diet. This usually means that the breastfed baby will be more accepting of new foods and flavours when the time comes to introduce solids.
- Finally, another effect (and benefit for some) is that high levels of prolactin suppress ovulation, which can prevent resumption of your periods and therefore delay the return of your fertility.

Benefits of breastfeeding for you

- It is convenient, with no need to make up formula feeds or clean up afterwards.
- It is less expensive – no need to buy artificial milks or purchase the accessories required for bottle-feeding.
- It helps you lose your pregnancy weight more quickly.
- There are fewer incidences of breast cancer, ovarian cancer, osteoporosis and post-partum depression in women who breastfeed.
- It may delay the return of your periods and ovulation.
- It has the potential to improve your diabetic control if you suffer with diabetes.
- You are likely to return to your optimal weight more easily.

Q. Are there any dangers in breast milk?

Because your milk contains anything you have taken in there may be some substances, such as cigarette smoke or caffeine, present in breast milk which could be passed on to the breastfeeding baby.

Cigarette smoking can reduce prolactin levels, which can affect the amount of breast milk produced. It can also affect oxytocin, so affecting your letdown reflex. It is therefore advisable for you to avoid smoking while you are breastfeeding.

You may have read or heard in the media about a variety of chemicals that could be passed on in your breast milk. Try not to worry about these, as they are usually chemicals that are naturally present in our water and diet, so your baby is at no greater risk just because you are breastfeeding.

Q. Should I avoid certain foods if I am breastfeeding?

You will probably hear that you should avoid spicy foods, or gas-producing foods such as Brussels sprouts, but this is not necessarily true – it will depend on your baby. Ideally you should include a wide variety of foods in your diet; anything and everything in moderation, unless you find, from experience, that eating a particular type of food really does seem to upset your baby. Eating a dozen oranges or lots of fruit juice may result in your baby having loose stools, but if you only eat one or two, or just a glass of juice then this is not likely to cause any problems.

It is probably a good idea to avoid alcohol, although an occasional glass won't be too harmful, although it is best if you leave two hours after having a drink before breastfeeding.

If you need to take any prescription medicines, you should ask your doctor if it is okay to continue with these while you are breastfeeding. Most 'over the counter' medicines, such as paracetamol, are likely to be okay for you to take occasionally, if you really need to, although there isn't any actual proof of this. Certain medicines, such as antihistamines, which may be in some medicines for allergy or even cough remedies, can cause you to become dehydrated, which in turn can affect the amount of milk you produce. Do always check the packet or literature for any medicine you take to check that it is suitable while breastfeeding. If you do need to take any medicines, try to breastfeed before taking the medication. You should avoid taking any 'recreational' drugs while breastfeeding.

Breastfeeding is the best thing you can do for your baby – breastfeed for as long as you can in order to maximize the benefits, but remember that breastfeeding for any length of time is better than not at all.

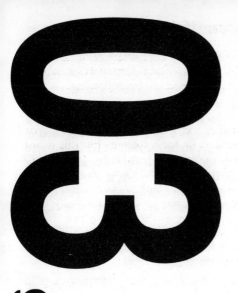

03

getting started

In this chapter you will learn:
- how to prepare yourself for breastfeeding
- what equipment you may need
- the best start to breastfeeding
- how to make sure your baby is positioned and attached correctly.

Preparing for breastfeeding

Q. Do I need to prepare my breasts for breastfeeding?

No, you really don't need to – nature does all the preparation for you. You will notice that your breasts change during pregnancy, with the area around your nipple (the areola) becoming darker. You do not need to roll or scrub your nipples to 'toughen them up' as may have been suggested in the past. It has no value and can be painful. Don't be tempted to apply anything that is too drying to your nipples; it is not necessary and may mean they become more, not less, likely to crack. Sometimes, even using soap to wash your breasts can be quite drying and mean your nipples are more likely to crack.

Your skin colour will have no influence on whether you experience sore nipples or not. This is down to correct positioning and 'latching-on' of your baby.

What you do need to do in preparation for breastfeeding is to ensure that you are armed with the facts and have made the positive decision to breastfeed. It may be useful to attend an antenatal session, held by your local midwife, where you can gather information. You may also find it useful to attend a local National Childbirth Trust (NCT) group or La Leche League group (see 'Taking it further'). This should provide you with all the information you need, and will also enable you to meet other mothers and mothers-to-be who can prove to be an essential support network later on.

It is also a good idea to look at your breasts and become familiar with them; touch them and get used to how they feel – where they feel lumpy and bumpy. Performing this routine regularly is a good habit to get into anyway, but particularly in relation to pregnancy and breastfeeding it will help you to know what is normal for you. You may notice some leaking of 'milk' from your breasts while pregnant, but you don't need to try and express anything.

Equipment you may need

There are a few pieces of equipment that you will find extremely useful when breastfeeding.

Nursing bras

Q. When should I be fitted for a bra?

I would suggest that you are fitted for a bra some time after you have reached 36 weeks. Ideally have a couple of nursing/maternity bras before you deliver. You may need to have another one or two once feeding is well under way, but it is wise to wait until you have settled down into breastfeeding before being fitted for these, to make sure you get the size you really need.

If you can, go to a specialist bra shop where they will be able to advise you on what you need. Make sure the bra allows for when your breasts increase in size as your milk comes in, as well as when they settle down and reduce in size after the first 12 weeks. The bra should have several rows of fasteners to give you that flexibility.

During pregnancy your breasts will have become a lot heavier, but they have little to support them so it is important to ensure you have a properly fitting bra and make sure the straps are wide enough not to cut into you while maintaining your support. While you are pregnant you will find that your breasts steadily increase in size, so you should try to be re-measured every six to eight weeks.

Useful tips for buying a bra

- Try buying maternity/nursing bras that unhook or unzip at the front as these are easier when trying to feed, rather than needing to unfasten your bra at the back. They will also continue to support your other breast during feeding.
- If you buy your bra late in pregnancy, make sure it feels comfortable when you fasten it on the last set of hooks, so when you have delivered and your ribcage has decreased in size it will still be comfortable and give you support.
- Try on several types of bra and try to undo them with just one hand to see how easy it is, as your other hand will usually be occupied holding your baby.
- Make sure the bra has wide straps and a broad band underneath the bust for good support and to eliminate 'bounce'.
- Try the bra on under different clothes to find out what types of clothing will be easier to wear – button-up shirts, T-shirts or specially designed 'nursing' clothes.
- It is best to avoid under-wired nursing bras as these can constrict the ducts in your breast and may lead to mastitis.

Breast pads

You will also need some breast pads. These can be washable or a disposable variety – try not to use those with a plastic backing regularly as these tend to make your nipples sweat and may lead to an increase in the likelihood of soreness. The machine-washable pads are better value in the long run but may not seem quite as convenient as disposable pads. You don't really need any creams or lotions to put on your nipples, although there are plenty on the market. If you do decide to use a cream, you should check on the package whether it needs to be washed off before feeding, and gradually reduce its use. Some women are sensitive to the ingredients in some of these creams, in particular lanolin, so if you do use such products you may find little improvement or even find your symptoms worsening.

Top tip

If you do experience some soreness you can express a little colostrum/milk and rub this around the nipples.

Sterilizing equipment

You may need sterilizing fluid and a container in which to sterilize equipment. This may be useful if you wish or need to express breast milk, especially if you are thinking of going back to work. Some small bottles/containers into which to express your breast milk are needed, or you may choose to use disposable plastic bags, which are available specifically for storing breast milk.

The container does not need to be a commercial 'sterilizing tank'; you could use any large plastic tub, for example an old clean ice-cream tub may be sufficient for your needs if you are not sterilizing a large number of bottles. This will be less costly both in terms of buying the equipment and also in terms of the quantity of sterilization fluid required for the size of container (as the commercial tanks can be large). You can use sterilizing liquid or tablets for cold sterilization, whichever you find easier. If you are not going to use the container regularly, it may be sufficient to use sterilizing tablets, just in case you need them. These may be more convenient to store and carry with you, especially if you are travelling, for example.

Breast pumps

Some women find breast pumps useful, although there is no real need for one. Most women can undertake hand expression, when taught correctly, which is far more convenient: there is nothing to wash and sterilize after use; your hands are more portable and only need to be washed before expressing begins. Your midwife should be able to assist in teaching you how to express your milk, although it is also covered later in this book.

Recap

Items you may find useful to prepare for breastfeeding:

- maternity/nursing bras that unfasten at the front
- breast pads – machine-washable or disposable
- plastic container to use as a sterilizer
- sterilizing fluid or tablets
- a couple of bottles or small containers into which to express breast milk – wide-necked bottles are much easier for this
- breast pump – not essential as hand expression is more effective and convenient
- creams/lotions/sprays – again not essential as expressed colostrum can be rubbed around the nipple and areola area and is more effective.

Skin-to-skin contact

An ideal way to get to know your new baby is through skin-to-skin contact. This is a lovely way for you and your new baby to get acquainted, and your partner could also share this experience.

Your midwife may deliver your baby directly on to your tummy, or may dry him off a little first and then place him on your tummy. She will then cover you both with a towel while you share this special time together. Skin-to-skin contact helps to keep your baby warm, as new babies have a tendency to lose heat when they are delivered, as they are still wet and the temperature of the room will be lower than that in your womb.

Skin-to-skin contact also helps to build up the bond between you and your baby. Where possible, this skin-to-skin contact should continue until you wish it to end, preferably after your baby has had his first breastfeed. Often skin-to-skin contact can lead to the baby breastfeeding – if left, your baby will start to crawl and make his own way to your breast (although this can take up to an hour). This is a very special time for both of you. Discuss this with your midwife during your pregnancy and ask her to write it into your 'birth plan' or make a record of your requests regarding this in your notes. Sometimes when maternity units are busy this can be overlooked or seem hurried, so don't be afraid to ask for this time together.

However, even if you don't want to breastfeed this should not stop you from experiencing this initial skin-to-skin contact as it will help you to feel closer to your baby. Babies find skin-to-skin contact very comforting as they can hear your heartbeat and feel your closeness. They also learn to recognize your scent, which becomes familiar and reassuring to them, so if your baby is unsettled this may help to comfort him. Mothers who use skin-to-skin contact do tend to breastfeed longer than those who do not.

'When I first thought of having my baby delivered and put straight onto my tummy I was not too keen. But when my midwife put him there, he just looked so calm; it was beautiful. We left him there and then he just started trying to crawl towards my breast – it was amazing!'

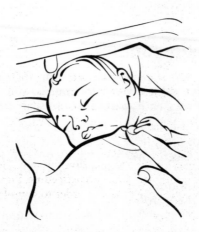

figure 3.1 skin-to-skin contact following delivery

Benefits of skin-to-skin contact

- It helps keep your baby warm.
- It can be calming for both you and your baby.
- It helps regulate your baby's heartbeat and breathing.
- It can help to stimulate your baby to search for and find your breast.
- It can help stimulate oxytocin release, which may help in reducing your blood loss after delivery.
- It can help improve weight gain in your baby.
- It helps foster your new relationship with your baby.

Skin-to-skin contact is not just useful in the early days but can be used any time. It can help calm your baby and may assist in encouraging your baby to feed if he does not seem very interested. Letting your baby have skin-to-skin contact will encourage him to nuzzle and search for your breast.

Your partner may also enjoy skin-to-skin contact to help develop his relationship with your new baby. Also, your partner can provide the skin-to-skin contact if, for instance, you are unable to hold your baby straight after delivery for any reason, for example if you have had a Caesarean section. Your partner can cuddle baby by putting him inside his shirt or even taking his shirt off if he prefers.

Your first feed

One of the next most important steps in breastfeeding your baby is his very first feed. Don't be afraid to ask your midwife to help you put your baby to the breast for the first time (at the very least). Even if you have breastfed a previous baby, don't be shy of asking for help – every baby is different. The sooner your baby can have his first breastfeed following birth the better; but if either of you is not well enough, don't worry! He will benefit whenever you are able to start breastfeeding him. If possible, you can express your breast milk in order to stimulate your milk supply.

If the first feed is difficult it can undermine your confidence and lead to further difficulties in later feeds. However, if you do have problems initially, don't panic – ask your midwife for assistance, as she should be able to help you get it right and you will then be more likely to breastfeed your baby for as long as you want to. If there is any reason why you cannot feed your baby (for example, if he is ill and needs specialist care), try to express your breast milk. There may not seem to be very much milk there but every little helps and it is very important. The milk you express at first will be colostrum, which will contain valuable nutrients and antibodies for your baby; and the act of expressing will help your body begin the process of milk production as it will stimulate the production of prolactin, the milk-producing hormone.

Q. I don't seem to have much milk. Is my baby getting enough?

A healthy newborn baby born at term often does not feed very frequently in the first couple of days – he should have sufficient stores of energy to last until your milk comes in (remember, this is when your mature breast milk production begins). So don't worry that you are not giving your baby enough – remember that colostrum is a very rich and concentrated substance containing protein, which is essential for growth and development. In the first 24 hours your baby only needs around $1\frac{1}{2}$ teaspoons of milk each feed, so the small amount of colostrum you produce will be ample.

Your feeding position

When putting your baby to the breast, make sure you are comfortable first. Try not to lean backwards or forwards. Sitting upright, supported by pillows is a good position if you are in bed. If you are sitting on a chair, make sure that it is comfortable and that your feet reach the floor, or put a stool (or some books) under them. Your legs (lap) should not be sloping down, nor should your legs be raised too high. If the chair is quite deep you may need to put some cushions or pillows behind you to ensure you are sitting upright. Don't be tempted to lean forward into your baby, to drop your breast into his mouth, as this may not be helpful for correct attachment, and it can be difficult for you to maintain this position throughout the feed. You will get tired and your back will ache. It is very important that you make sure you are comfortable before you start to feed so that you can relax and allow letdown to happen.

Another option is to lie on your side and bring your baby into you. Keep your baby's head, shoulders and spine all in one line;

don't just turn the baby's head. Think how uncomfortable you would feel if you tried to eat or drink while turning your head. Bring your baby into you, mostly chest to chest – your tummy and his tummy should be in contact; to do this the baby will need to be lying on his side. If your breasts are larger and point downwards rather than straight ahead, it can help if your baby is lying facing slightly upwards, but do remember to keep the head and spine all in one line, not twisted at all. You can then support the head and shoulders. Don't restrict movement of your baby's head by holding it at the back, in case he needs to move it. Place your hand behind the shoulders instead. This position is discussed in more detail below.

> **Top tip**
>
> It often helps to bring your baby slowly towards your breast from the centre of your body, rather than straight towards your nipple ('front-on'), which seems more like aiming for the target rather than allowing your baby to come in slowly. It also gives you time to adjust your baby's position.

You then need to 'tease' the baby with your nipple. Baby's nose and top lip should be in line with your nipple at this point, so when baby does open his mouth wide this will ensure the nipple goes towards the back and upper part of the mouth. Then, by brushing the nipple downwards towards his mouth you will encourage your baby to 'gape' – usually he will naturally tilt his head back first and then open his mouth.

Holding your baby

You may need to experiment with different ways of holding your baby (see below) until you feel completely comfortable. This will depend upon how you and your baby fit together or whether you find it easier feeding from one breast more than the other. Often, if you are right handed, it seems easier to feed on the left breast as there is some uncertainty 'where to put your hands' when trying to feed on the right side.

Make sure you are not holding the back of your baby's head as this will prevent him from opening his mouth wide and latching on properly. You can hold your breast by cupping your hand underneath it with your thumb and fingers in a 'C' shape.

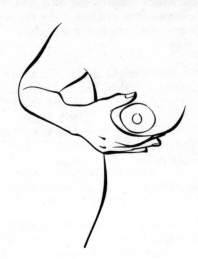

figure 3.2 hand cupping breast in a 'C' shape

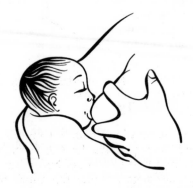

figure 3.3 the scissor hold

Don't use a 'scissor-hold' (spreading two fingers around the nipple) as this can result in either pulling the nipple back or restricting the flow of milk through the ducts.

Don't be in a hurry to put your baby on to the breast at this point; make sure his tongue is down and covering the lower gums before pulling his bottom in towards you and attaching him to your breast. If this doesn't happen straight away, don't worry – he will learn how wide he needs to open his mouth. Be patient, take him away and start again until his mouth is wide open, like a yawn! His tongue should be down and formed ready to 'scoop' the breast tissue. As he goes to the breast his lips should be rolled back, exposing the gums ready to latch firmly on to the breast tissue, as shown in Figure 3.4a. Figure 3.4b shows the baby at the breast well attached.

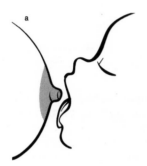 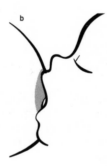

figure 3.4 a) Baby with a wide gape about to go to the breast   b) Well-attached baby with a wide gape

Don't worry if it takes your baby a few attempts at this; you are both learning and, with practice, he will learn how wide he needs to open his mouth. It should not hurt when your baby is attached correctly, although you may feel a little tender if your nipples have already become sore.

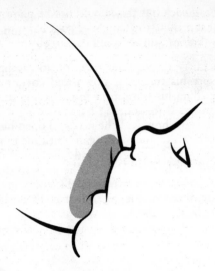

figure 3.5 poorly attached baby – mouth is not open wide enough ('prissy lips')

Once your baby is suckling there should not be any pain, if there is you need to take him off the breast (put your little finger in the corner of his mouth to 'break the seal') and try again. Once your baby is attached properly, look at the amount of your areola (the pink/brown area around the nipple) you can see; you will probably still be able to see some at the top. If you can't, don't worry, you may have a smaller areola. The amount you can see will not necessarily be even all round as your baby will not take the same amount of areola tissue from the top and bottom of the nipple into his mouth – he should take more of the lower areola into his mouth. Your baby's chin should be lying against your breast if he is correctly positioned. There may only be a small gap between your breast and your baby's nose, but don't be tempted to try to indent your breast with your hand to 'make space' for your baby to breathe; this can constrict the milk ducts and restrict your milk flow.

If your baby is latched on well you should notice that following his initial rapid sucks there is a change to slower, deeper sucks with pauses as he swallows. Don't think baby has stopped feeding; this is quite normal. You may be aware that your baby has quite a strong suck but this should not be painful. You may notice movement around the temple of your baby, as his muscles move, or some babies 'wiggle' their ears. You may also be able to hear swallowing sounds, although in the first few days the amount your baby will be swallowing is so small that any swallowing may be infrequent and fairly quiet. Your baby's cheeks should be full, and not sucked in, as this would suggest he is not latched on quite correctly.

Good attachment – what to look for

- Have baby's top lip in line with your nipple.
- Ensure baby is turned to face you – chest to chest or tummy to tummy.
- His head and spine should be in one straight line, not twisted.
- Hold your baby in close to you, well supported with your hands and pillows as needed.
- Don't let his head tilt down; the head should be straight.
- His lips will be rolled back and his tongue down.
- Baby's mouth should be wide open – as his mouth opens, his head will tilt backwards.
- Baby's cheeks will be full and rounded – there should be no dimpling.
- You may not be able to see much, if any, of the areola – although more of the underside than upper part should be in your baby's mouth.
- If supporting your breast, cup your hand underneath and form a 'C' shape with your thumb and fingers – don't distort the shape of your breast.
- Baby's chin should be in close to your breast; there may only be a small gap between your breast and baby's nose but don't pull your breast back to create a gap.

Once baby is attached you need to make sure your position is comfortable and sustainable for the duration of the feed. So you may need to put a pillow under baby's bottom for support, for example, or under your arm.

Breastfeeding positions

There are a number of different positions you can try, which are discussed below.

'Cradle' hold

You may need to use pillows/cushions under baby's bottom to bring him up to your breast at the right height, so you don't have to lean forward.

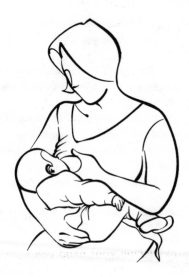

figure 3.6 'Cradle' hold

When in this position, put baby's lower arm around your waist towards your back. His head should be resting in the bend of your arm, your arm supporting his back and your hand supporting his bottom. Use your other hand to 'cup' and offer the other breast.

'Rugby/football' hold

You may need cushions behind you as well as under baby as he lies on, or under, your arm. This position can be helpful if you are feeding twins, although you may need some help initially to get both babies on the breast simultaneously. It is also a good position as your baby grows, as there is more room for his legs, under your arms.

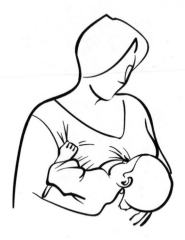

figure 3.7 'Rugby/football' hold

Support your baby by placing your hand behind his neck, with his back resting along your arm. Use the other hand to offer him your breast.

Lying on your side in bed

This position has already been introduced above. It is often a good position, especially the first few times you breastfeed, while you are still in hospital. It is also good for feeding during the night, or when you are having a rest.

Make sure you are lying completely on your side and baby is feeding from the 'lower' breast. As mentioned earlier, turn baby completely towards you and bring him in close to you. You may find it comfortable to put your lower arm above your head or rest on it.

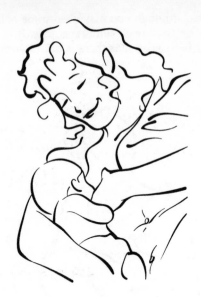

figure 3.8 lying on your side to feed

It can be difficult to turn over to feed from the other side, especially if you have had a Caesarean section or have painful stitches. In this case, you can remain lying on the same side and lay your baby on a pillow to bring him up to the level of the upper breast; then lean/roll further in towards your baby so you can feed using the 'upper' breast.

'Cross-cradle' hold

This uses the arm opposite to the breast being used to feed from to support the baby, unlike the cradle hold where the baby lies on the arm so the head is supported in the crook of the arm. Again make sure your hand is not holding baby's head, but supporting him at the back of his shoulders. It will probably still be helpful to put a pillow under baby to raise him up, rather than you feeling you have to lean into him.

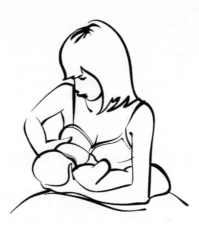

figure 3.9 'Cross-cradle' hold

Each of these positions may be useful for you at different times, for example if you are too sore to sit comfortably initially, then lying on your side may be better for you in the early days. Obviously this will be less convenient when you are up and about and out shopping!

Many women feel more comfortable putting their baby on one particular side; in this case it may be useful to vary the hold depending upon which side he is feeding from. You may find you prefer the cradle or cross-cradle hold when feeding on your left breast, especially if you are right handed, as this hand will be supporting your baby. However, when swapping to the right breast you may feel unsure about where to put your hands, so try the rugby-ball hold. You may need a pillow on that side to support baby's bottom but, essentially, you are then treating your right breast as if it were on the left side.

Once your baby is on your breast, relax and let your shoulders drop. Uncurl your toes, which you may find are quite tense. Now ask yourself, 'Does it hurt?' After the initial attachment there should be no pain. If it does hurt there's a good chance the positioning is not quite right; it may only need minor adjustment but this may be vital to your comfort and a successful feed. Ask your midwife to watch you and then she will be able to determine what, if any, adjustments are needed. As already mentioned, your midwife should be available to help you with your very first feed, although if this is not your first baby you may not feel this is necessary. However, every baby is different so don't feel you should know what to do. Ask for any help you can.

How to know when your baby is hungry

In the first couple of days your baby may not feed very frequently; some babies may only feed three or four times in the first 24 hours, but the frequency will normally increase after this. This is why 'baby-led' feeding (i.e. feeding your baby when he is hungry) is so important. When your baby wakes or shows signs of wanting to feed you need to recognise his feeding 'cues' – you should then be ready to breastfeed him.

The cues to look for

When your baby first wakes he will be in a quiet but alert stage. He will then often start 'rooting' (searching for the breast) and snuffling, perhaps trying to find his fist. He may make sucking type actions and if he can find his hand he may start sucking on that.

As he progresses through these stages he will become more 'fussy' and there will be more movement of both arms and legs. If these stages are ignored then he may become more tense and only then will he cry for his feed.

You should aim to recognize these feeding cues as early as possible, rather than waiting for him to start crying. Once he starts crying attachment becomes more difficult and this tends to result in a windier baby, as he will take a lot of air into his stomach when he is crying. Try to stay calm; this can be difficult when your baby is so unsettled, but if you are also agitated your baby will sense this and become more upset. You will learn to recognize when your baby needs feeding as you become more attuned to his behaviour.

As your baby grows older and becomes more accustomed to breastfeeding you may find he opens his mouth and sticks out his tongue, in a scoop-shape. He may increase how often he does this, sticking his tongue out further and further until you finally respond and breastfeed him.

Feeding cues

Your baby may:

- be wakeful, quiet but alert
- start 'rooting' and snuffling around
- find his fist and start sucking on that
- make sucking actions – older babies may stick out their tongue in anticipation
- become increasingly 'fussy'
- increase his hand, arm and leg movements
- have a tense posture
- finally start crying.

Where to feed

In the early days – the first couple of weeks or so – try to feed in a calm environment. This may be difficult as you will probably find you have lots of visitors. However, it is important to find the time and space for you and your baby to get together, as this will help build up your confidence and increase how well you can 'latch him on'. You need to ensure that neither you nor your baby are distracted. If you are surrounded by lots of visitors you may feel uncomfortable about feeding him in front of them, which may lead you to try to placate your baby by letting him suck your finger or cuddling/rocking instead of responding to the early feeding cues. While this may succeed in soothing him temporarily, it will also prolong the time between feeds, which in turn will have an effect on the amount of milk you produce. If the time between feeds is too long your milk will not be stimulated frequently enough and so less will be produced.

Similarly, if you feel embarrassed you may rush the feed and not take that little extra time needed in those early days to ensure that your baby is attached properly. If he is not attached correctly this could lead to sore nipples and thus to pain for you, when feeding, which makes it less likely that you attach your baby properly at the next feed because it hurts. This can then become a vicious cycle.

If you do have lots of visitors, maybe your partner could talk to them while you feed the baby, or perhaps you could stagger the numbers or arrange for them to visit at different times, when you are less likely to be feeding. This can be difficult to predict in the early days, which is often the time when your friends and family want to see you and your new arrival. If necessary, you could always go to your bedroom to breastfeed, although this may make you feel quite isolated. However, once you are more confident in attaching your baby to the breast you will probably find that you are able to feed him more discreetly, so do not need to take yourself off somewhere private to feed. Also bear in mind that your visitors will understand if you need to go and feed your baby, and will probably appreciate that when you have fed him he will be more settled.

But before we look in more detail at the day-to-day feeding arrangements once you are both home, let's look at the issues that may arise in the first few feeds.

04

the early days in hospital

In this chapter you will learn:
- how often to feed your baby in the early days
- what can stop you from feeding well in the early days
- how hospital routines impact on you and your baby.

Starting out

This chapter is intended to help you during the first couple of days after giving birth, especially if you are in hospital, as this may influence how you cope with feeding your new baby.

The time you spend in hospital following your delivery will vary depending upon where you have your baby. In most cases you will probably have your baby in hospital and in some cases you may be able to stay in for about four days following your delivery. But in many hospitals it is becoming more likely that you will be encouraged to go home much earlier. In some cases, if both you and your baby are well, you may be able to go home within 24 hours of the birth. You may be lucky enough to have had a home birth, in which case you will be at home anyway. If so, you will need to make sure you have some support at home for the few days after the birth so that you can rest and recover.

There are some advantages to staying in hospital for few days, for example, you may be able to get more help when you need it from the midwives and hospital staff; but it can also be more difficult to settle into your own routine. If you are at home you can have everything close to hand, but it will mean that if you have any worries you either have to wait for your midwife to visit or you will have to telephone someone.

Q. When should I start to breastfeed?

Ideally you should attempt to feed your baby within the first hour after his birth; this is likely to increase your success at breastfeeding.

While in hospital, and especially for the first feed, you should ask your midwife for her help. As already mentioned, you may not stay in hospital for long, possibly for as little as 24 to 48 hours. Even if you have a more complicated delivery, such as forceps or Caesarean section, you may only be in hospital for about four to six days, depending on your local maternity unit. However long you are in hospital for, it is important that while you are there you use the staff and midwives available to gain as much support, advice and help from them as possible to make sure you are happy with caring for your baby and breastfeeding. It is to be hoped that you will have successfully carried out skin-to-skin contact following delivery and that your baby will have been to the breast for an uninterrupted feed. Feeding your baby soon after birth helps to release the milk-producing hormone prolactin, and the sooner this happens the better, as it helps 'prime' the cells in your breast that are responsible for secreting the milk. The more of these cells that are 'primed', the greater the potential amount of milk you are likely to be able to produce overall. Also, the more often your baby feeds the more often prolactin is released and so the greater the supply of milk produced.

Frequency of feeds

Q. How often should I feed my baby?

Ideally your baby should take about three or four feeds in his first 24 hours. Many babies are quite sleepy in the hours following their birth, so this is another good reason to try to feed your baby for as long as he wants as soon as possible after birth, as he may then sleep for some time. The frequency and number of feeds will increase around your third/fourth day when your milk 'comes in'.

You really need to put your baby to the breast as soon as practically possible, and then whenever he shows any interest in feeding. So if he starts sucking or mouthing his hands or is rooting for the nipple, you should be ready to let him breastfeed. Look at the feeding cues listed in Chapter 03.

If your baby has been to the breast shortly after delivery you may find he then sleeps for quite a long period and, if he is healthy and full term, this is nothing to worry about. However, when you are in hospital, you may be recommended to try to wake your baby for a feed. This may not be very successful as your baby may not really be interested at this time and attempting to feed him in this situation can be very frustrating and could undermine your future confidence.

In the first couple of days you should attempt to feed your baby at both breasts, as this will increase your levels of the hormone prolactin and therefore your milk supply. It is vitally important that you ensure that your baby is latched on and positioned correctly during these early days. For the first few days your baby will not get a great deal of milk (colostrum at this stage), but use this time to make sure you get your positioning right without worrying too much that your baby isn't getting enough milk.

Q. Should I take my baby off the breast when I think he's had enough?

It is not a good idea to take your baby off the breast and it is not usually necessary, providing he is well positioned and attached properly. When he has finished, normally and ideally, he will come off the breast spontaneously and will then probably sleep for at least an hour and hopefully two to three.

During the first day your baby may sleep more between feeds, not necessarily waking every two hours; if you have had any pethidine during labour then your baby is likely to be sleepier during the first couple of days. Remember, if your baby went to the breast soon after delivery and had a good feed, he may sleep for several hours on your first day. A newborn can spend more than 60% of his time sleeping.

If your baby needs to feed more frequently than two-hourly in the first couple of days, and these feeds are taking as long as an hour, you will need to make sure that he is positioned and latched on correctly, as it may be that he is not getting enough milk (colostrum). Ask your midwife to look at your positioning and check the attachment when you are feeding your baby.

table 4.1 frequency of breastfeeds for your baby

Age of your baby	Frequency of feeding
Baby in first 24 hours	Infrequent; may be as few as three feeds in the first 24 hours.
Under 7 days	Will increase in frequency, especially around days 4 to 5. May have as many as 12 feeds per day during this time.
Over 7 days	Will continue to feed frequently, as many as eight feeds per day, often in 'clusters'.

Your baby may not fall asleep immediately after feeding (although a lot of time is spent sleeping between feeds), but may spend a little time alert and just looking at you. This is a lovely time for cuddles; don't worry about spoiling him. He has been close to you and heard your heartbeat for nine months and this closeness is very comforting for him.

Q. Do I need to wind my baby after a breastfeed?

No, generally breastfed babies tend to bring up their wind when you sit them up, or pass it through the other end! Occasionally after a feed you may notice that baby's top lip looks a little darker in colour, which usually means he does have some wind. In this case, sit him upright, supporting his back so his gullet is straight and this will allow him to bring up any 'trapped' wind. However, you will get used to your baby and will know whether or not he tends to be 'windy'.

Q. What could prevent a successful 'early' feed?

If your delivery was subject to any interventions such as a Caesarean section, or if you or your baby are too tired to feed immediately following delivery, then you may not be able to have a successful attempt at feeding after your delivery. If you have not managed to have a good feed at delivery, don't worry – all is not lost! Worrying in itself will have a negative effect on your breastfeeding, as worry and anxiety inhibit the flow of the hormone oxytocin, which is necessary for your 'letdown'.

Q. What should I do if my baby is very sleepy?

Your baby maybe very sleepy following delivery, particularly if you have had pain relief during your labour. If this is the case, you will need either to stimulate him to feed regularly or to express your breasts every couple of hours and collect the colostrum. This will stimulate your hormonal response to release prolactin and so to produce milk.

If your baby is well but just sleepy during the first day, let your midwife know, but try to express your breast milk every couple of hours until your baby is awake to feed.

Top tip

If your baby is sleepy, express some breast milk while waiting for him to wake. This expressed milk can be used if there are times when you feel your baby needs more milk.

Amount of milk consumed

During the first few days you will produce colostrum, and your baby will not usually need any large volumes of this type of milk – about 1½ teaspoons per feed on the first day, rising to about 15 ml (a large tablespoonful) on the second day and then to around 1 ounce on the third day – when the breast milk will normally start to come in. So, although your baby does not need huge amounts of colostrum, you do need to stimulate the supply so that milk production is not delayed. If you do not put your baby to the breast regularly (or express your breasts) then you will not be ready to produce the larger amounts when it is expected, as there will be some delay in your milk 'coming in'.

Q How will I know if my baby is getting sufficient milk?

Your baby should have wet nappies and the urine should not be dark and concentrated. If you are happy that this is happening then you can be sure your baby is getting enough milk. If there are no wet nappies or the urine is dark and concentrated you need to speak to your midwife as he may become dehydrated.

It is important to recognize the difference between a baby who does not need a feed and one that has tried to feed unsuccessfully. If you need to stimulate your baby to feed, remember to try skin-to-skin contact. The physical contact and nearness to you, together with your smell, will often encourage him to root for the breast and show interest in feeding.

If your baby becomes very hungry and starts to cry it can be difficult to put him straight to the breast as he will be too upset to settle into suckling. This will then lead to you becoming upset, making feeding more difficult. Instead, try to console him first, perhaps by using skin-to-skin contact. Talking to him gently and having eye contact with him can also help to calm him down. Then, when he is calmer, try again to breastfeed. It may be possible to avoid this situation altogether by being aware of 'hunger cues' (see Chapter 03) and, as your baby becomes more awake and alert, you can then be ready for him to feed. Of course, there will be times when this is not possible so don't feel a failure if your baby cries – but remember, not all cries mean 'Feed me!'

If your baby is not interested in feeding and seems jittery or jumpy then you may find your midwife is a little concerned and may wish to perform a blood test to check his sugar (glucose) levels. Depending upon the test results you may be advised to try to feed your baby more to increase his glucose and energy levels; if there is any concern the paediatrician (baby doctor) will be informed.

Q. Do I need to feed from both breasts?

During these first few days you should expect to feed your baby from both breasts at each feed, alternating which side you start on. When you have been breastfeeding and your baby comes off on his own, sit him up, and if he still seems interested and awake, then it is likely he will need to go on the other breast too. When it comes to the next feed, put your baby on whichever side you finished the last feed on. If your baby only takes one breast at each feed then feed from the other breast at the next feed. You may read or hear advice that baby only needs one breast at each feed, and this can be true for some babies, but not usually in the first few days. This may change once your milk supply is more established.

Feeds in the first few days will be relatively short as baby receives only small volumes of colostrum at each feed. If your feeds are taking longer than half an hour in the first few days you need to check that he is correctly attached as incorrect latching on can make for long ineffective feeds. Also, if your baby is not attached correctly you are more likely to experience sore nipples.

If your baby is not really suckling but just lying with your nipple in his mouth, then there is no need to leave him there. Try not to let him just lie asleep with your nipple in his mouth. This can lead to you becoming sore. Usually babies will come off the breast on their own, if they have been attached correctly, and will then settle well. In the first few weeks of your baby's life he will feed and sleep and do little else.

A normal feed will include some 'non-nutritive' sucking – these are short sucks without swallowing and usually happen at the start of the feed. This helps stimulate the letdown reflex (and oxytocin release) and the milk flow. Many babies have a period of 'cluster feeding' associated with increased wakefulness at around 20–24 hours of age. This will often follow a time of deep sleep after an initial eagerness to feed within the first couple of hours following delivery.

Your milk supply will be mainly colostrum in the first couple of days, which is a concentrated substance so doesn't need to be produced in large volumes. The baby's stomach is only quite small and doesn't need to take in large volumes at this stage. The following table demonstrates the small quantities of milk baby takes in the first few days and how these increase after the time when your milk will have come in (usually around day 3 or 4).

table 4.2 breast milk production from birth

Age of baby	Volume per day		Volume per feed
	Range	Average	On average
Day 1 (0–24 hours)	7–123 ml	37 ml	7 ml
Day 2 (24–48 hrs)	44–335 ml	84 ml	14 ml
Day 3 (48–72 hrs)	98–775 ml	408 ml	38 ml
Day 4 (72–96 hrs)	375–876 ml	625 ml	58 ml
Day 5 (95–120 hrs)	452–876 ml	700 ml	70 ml

Adapted from RCM (Inch & Woolridge, 1995)

Q. Can I give any extra milk to my baby?

Providing your baby wakes for feeding, then feeds well and takes himself off the breast, it is not necessary to give him any extra milk. If your baby is very sleepy and jaundiced he may need to be given more milk. But if this is the case then it is better if you can express your breast milk and then feed this milk to him.

If you are having problems, with baby refusing to latch on and you are unable to get him to feed at your breast, then express your breast milk as often as you can. Ideally the expressed milk should be cup fed to your baby, but cup feeding can be a bit of a messy business, especially if your baby is healthy, hungry and full term, so use a bib or napkin around him when feeding in this way. It is easier to cup feed in the first few days, usually because there are only small volumes involved. When larger volumes are being given it can be quite slow as well as messy. If you can cup feed, great, but if this is not working for you then give the expressed milk in a bottle. It is better that your baby has expressed breast milk from a bottle than has no breast milk at all.

Q. *How do I give my baby expressed breast milk?*

It is better to try and use a cup rather than giving your baby a bottle as this may cause confusion when you then try to put your baby back on the breast. The action baby uses to feed from the teat on a bottle is very different from feeding from the breast and if your baby gets used to feeding from a bottle he may be less inclined to put in the extra effort to 'milk' the breast. However, the action of the tongue used when cup feeding is similar to that when breastfeeding (rather like a kitten 'lapping') and this can help your baby to feed at the breast successfully.

Q. *Do I need to use a special cup when trying to cup feed milk to my baby?*

You should use a small cup with a lip around the rim, not a hard edge as this has to rest against the baby's mouth. A small 'medicine tot' or even a small egg-cup would be suitable for this. These can also be sterilized easily between feeds. The level of milk in the 'cup' needs to be close to the top so that when it is put to the baby's mouth he can lap at the milk; you should not attempt to pour the milk into the mouth.

Once your breastfeeding is established you can occasionally give your baby expressed breast milk via a bottle. For example, if there are times when you wish to leave your baby while you go out it is possible for your childminder/partner/babysitter to give your breast milk in this way.

Settling into a routine

One of the problems you may have while you are in hospital is trying to establish a routine – maternity wards have a routine of their own and this may not fit in with you and or your baby. Sometimes the midwife or a doctor will want to examine you or your baby and this may not always coincide with you or him being awake. Also, you are very likely to be in a ward area with other mothers and babies. This is very useful for support and to help you to make friends and contacts for the future – you have a lot in common and this is often a starting point to building up your new social network. However, because you are sharing with other babies and mothers, who will probably have a different routine from yours, this means that while you are hoping to rest another baby may be awake and wanting to feed, so it can sometimes be difficult to rest adequately. On the positive side, you will see how other breastfed babies behave. They are unlikely all to behave in the same way and this can highlight to you the importance of baby-led feeding. On the down side, if you are sharing a ward with mostly bottle-feeding mothers and babies this can lead to you feeling a little isolated and disheartened as they seem to sleep so much longer between feeds (in the early days) than your breastfeeding baby. Just remember why this is – look back at the differences in the composition of breast milk compared with bottled milk, and the size of baby's stomach, discussed in Chapter 02. Try not to worry about it and just accept that it won't last forever, and remember that those regular feeds are really helpful in building up your milk supply.

Q. *Why won't my baby sleep through the night?*

In the early days your breastfeeding baby is unlikely to sleep through the night. In fact this is good for breastfeeding, although you may not agree in the middle of the night.

Night feeds are really helpful in building up your milk supply, as the hormone response is much greater during the night. This can also lead to feelings of isolation, especially if no one else seems to be awake but you; it sometimes feels like the whole world is asleep except you! But the result of these night feeds is that your prolactin levels surge to ten times the amount they would during a day feed – this is really good news for your milk supply. The higher the prolactin levels, the more milk you make. It may be because you are more rested, but whatever the reason, seize these opportunities.

Remember to try to rest during the day to recover, especially if you have been up during the night, otherwise you will soon start to feel exhausted. This can be at its worst around day 3 or 4, when you tend to be a bit low anyway as the excitement of the birth gives way to the drop in hormones. This is often referred to as 'baby blues' and is quite normal, so do not worry if you are a bit tearful. However, if you are also losing sleep and feel you are having problems feeding this can all seem too much, so do try and rest as often as you can – when your baby is sleeping, you should try to do the same.

Hospital and visitors

Another problem that can result from being in hospital is that there are often lots of other people around, hospital routines to fit in with and visitors (yours or other people's) who may also disturb you when you are trying to rest. Your visitors in particular, although welcome, may not appreciate your need for rest. Everyone wants to see you and your new arrival and it can be difficult to manage the visiting schedule – although sometimes this can be just as bad when you are at home. But in hospital the problem may be other people's visitors. Many maternity hospitals now have a policy promoting 'open visiting', at least as far as the father of the baby is concerned. So your partner may be present in the ward for a large part of the day, but so may other people's partners. This may make you feel embarrassed about feeding in front of them. If so, check whether there is a special room where you can go to feed your baby – some maternity units do have these on the wards. If not, and you are still feeling a little awkward and need help getting baby to the breast, don't feel worried about drawing the curtains around your bed, which can afford you some much-needed privacy; and don't be upset if other mothers do the same when your partner is visiting.

Feeding during visiting time – Amy's experience

Amy was breastfeeding her first baby, Alice, but felt very awkward about breastfeeding in front of her visitors, especially when these included her father-in-law. If Alice cried for a feed while she had visitors, Amy would try to delay this feed. Often this meant Alice was passed around as each visitor tried to pacify her. When the visitors left and Amy attempted to breastfeed, Alice was often very difficult to settle and put on the breast.

I advised Amy that delaying the feed was actually causing Alice more upset, which then meant that she was too frustrated to attempt to feed. My suggestion was that Amy should attempt to feed Alice whenever she demanded it. Because Amy felt very self-conscious about feeding in public I advised her to look out for hunger cues that would allow her to anticipate the need for a feed a little earlier. This could then give Amy the chance to find somewhere to feed where she would feel comfortable. While breastfeeding, I suggested that Amy dressed cleverly, using shirts or tops with a hidden opening at the front in order that she didn't feel she had to 'display everything' when feeding.

While in hospital I suggested that Amy either pull the curtains around her bed, if there were other visitors in the area, or use the breastfeeding room that was available. Once at home, I suggested that Amy should take herself off to another room if visitors were in the house.

Q. Should there be a pattern to my baby's feeds?

In these early days you may feel your baby's feeding pattern is quite unpredictable, but go with it. Feed him when he wakes, for as long as he wants, until he literally drops off. Just ensure that his position is good and that he is attached properly at the breast, otherwise you will develop soreness.

It can be difficult to cope with establishing a breastfeeding routine alongside getting yourself sorted into a general routine and coping with new motherhood, but try not to put yourself under too much pressure. Where possible, relax; go with your baby's needs. This may not always be possible – sometimes you will have deadlines to meet, for example if you have other children there may be school collection times – but don't make things too problematic for yourself. Enlist as much assistance as you can to help you through this demanding time.

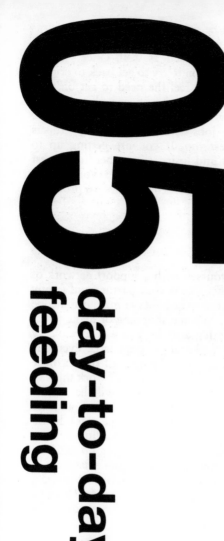

05

day-to-day feeding

In this chapter you will learn:
- the importance of getting help and setting up a routine
- about sleeping routines and night feeding
- how to maintain your lactation
- the best way to express your breast milk
- how to breastfeed your adoptive baby
- how to look after your baby if he was preterm
- how to look after your twins.

Breastfeeding your baby can be tiring. You will need to get as much rest as possible; if your baby is sleeping, take the opportunity to get some rest yourself as well. Once you are home there is always the temptation to try to get back to normal – whatever that means. You may feel the need to get on with housework and other jobs around the house, as well as looking after yourself and your new baby. However, you mustn't be tempted to try to fit in other jobs while he is sleeping – this is valuable time for you to rest too. If you are getting up to breastfeed through the night and losing sleep, then try to rest and recover this during the day. Don't feel guilty – you need to rest or you will become exhausted, which may lead to problems in feeding.

Getting help and rest

It is important to surround yourself with a support network of people who can help – whether this is your partner and family or good friends. You do not need to be Superwoman; if someone offers to collect the children, do some shopping or make you a cup of tea, accept the offer with gratitude. You will have plenty of opportunity to show how well you can cope later. Everyone likes to feel useful and you can make the most of this in those early days. If your partner can have some time off work this can help you and the family as a whole as you will have time together. Alternatively, your mother, mother-in-law or another relative may be willing and able to come and give you a hand. If this is during the day they may also be able do a little ironing and tidying up. These jobs have a way of building up and you may not be able to doing everything. Maybe a good friend could help with other children, perhaps with the school run, at least until you can predict your feeding pattern a little more. This sort of help is particularly important during the first couple of weeks while you are developing your own routine.

As a breastfeeding mother you are also helping to reduce your own workload, as there are no bottles to make up or to wash. Going out can take a lot of planning – making sure you take enough nappies, change of clothes etc. – so if you have one thing less to worry about, like bottles, trips can become a little easier.

Top tip

A good idea is to pack a 'travel bag' ready for these outings, containing all the items you may need: nappies, cotton wool, travel wipes and a barrier cream. You could prepare this before you have your baby, or when you first come home. It is much easier simply to add supplies to it after a trip out rather than having to start from scratch every time.

Remember, in the past the 'lying-in' period was meant to be just that, a period when the mother rested in bed for a length of time, to make sure she didn't overdo things. This lasted for up to ten days after delivery, although it was not necessarily good for new mothers because this can impact on circulation, for example. However, nowadays it seems that trends have moved to the other extreme. We often feel we have to be up within hours of delivery and this is not necessarily any better for us.

During the first week, try not to worry if you don't seem to make it out of your nightdress or pyjamas. If you find you can get dressed by lunchtime, see this as a bonus. This time should be a period of rest for you and your baby. If you have gone home within the first day or two after birth, which is increasingly common, be sure not to overdo things at home. Often you will find you are tearful and have the 'baby blues' around the fourth day and, if you are tired from not resting and undertaking night feeds, this can heighten these feelings.

Coping with visitors

Q. Lots of my friends and family want to visit. How can I get into a routine with so many visitors?

One of the consequences of being at home is that all your friends and relations will have the opportunity to pop round and see the new arrival. Lovely as this is, it can be very tiring for both of you. You will be unable to rest when you need to – not many visitors are comfortable about 'popping' round and then offering to make a cup of tea. You may feel you should be the polite hostess. Resist! If they do offer to make the tea, encourage them.

Another problem during these early days is that you are trying to get into some sort of routine and this can be easily disrupted. If visitors do come, usually they want to see baby, preferably awake, which may mean baby doesn't sleep when he needs to. He is likely to become increasingly fractious and unsettled and then it can take some time to get back into a less disruptive pattern. In the first couple of weeks it is likely that your baby may be sleeping when your visitors arrive, which also means their visit stops you from taking your much-needed rest.

Top tip

- Aim to have a rest at a given time of day.
- Take the phone off the hook.
- Turn your mobile off or on to silent – friends can leave a message and you can ring them to arrange a more convenient time to see them.
- Perhaps you could pre-arrange how long visitors should stay – or ask your partner to gently mention to them (maybe as they arrive) that you do need some rest. Visitors may not realize they are overstaying their welcome, and may in fact be worried to leave in case you feel they didn't want to come to start with.

Sleep patterns

The daytime nap

Q. Where should my baby sleep?

When you put your baby down to sleep for a nap, you need to consider where this should be. During the day it is a good idea to let him sleep in a Moses basket, carrycot or similar in the living room, close to you. This helps with feeding but also helps your baby start to notice the difference between night-time and daytime; this can help when trying to establish a routine for your baby's sleep pattern.

If your baby is having his nap nearby you can ensure that he does not need anything, and you can also pick up on 'feeding cues' that you might otherwise miss, which could result in the next feed being delayed so your baby is more fractious to put to the breast. You will come to learn what each of your baby's cries means. Take note of what else your baby is doing just before the crying starts. For example, is he rooting (searching for the breast)? These cues help you decide what the cries mean.

Q. What is 'rooting'?

Your newborn baby will turn his mouth, open and ready to suckle, towards any stimulus, such as when you stroke his cheek. This helps him find your breast ready for suckling. If you are holding your baby he can also smell you and your milk and this will help this reflex. This reflex tends to last until about three or four months.

Once you have fed your baby he may need a little 'activity' time. This will include nappy changing and perhaps a little play time associated with this. If your baby falls off the breast asleep, don't try to wake him, just let him sleep. As he grows and gets closer to two months of age he will be awake for longer after feeds so there will be more time for these activities. But the most important point to remember is to feed your baby when he wakes, and let him finish and come off the breast of his own accord. Do not take him off the breast, unless this is to adjust his position at the nipple.

Q. If my baby is taking his nap downstairs, should I keep quiet in case I wake him?

No, don't worry about household noise – young babies get used to this very quickly. For instance, if you have the radio on this is very unlikely to disturb him. It is better for you if he does get used to sleeping through some of the usual household noises, otherwise you may have a problem when you want to turn on the vacuum cleaner. Remember that for the last nine months he has heard muffled household sounds, so some of these may be comforting. Sudden loud noises, such as a harsh ring tone on your phone or doorbell, may disturb some babies, while for others this is not a problem. It really does depend on your baby – how sensitive he is. But trying to keep noise to an absolute minimum is not helpful as this prevents him from becoming used to a background 'hum'.

It is often recommended that you try to differentiate between day and night for your baby. Keeping him downstairs during the day gives the message that nights are for longer sleep, and this becomes associated with darkened quieter environments.

At around a month old you may find your baby is sleeping a little less during the day – take advantage of this and play with him and talk to him. As he gets older, at around three months or so, you might wish to let him have his afternoon nap in the bedroom, which may ensure he is less disturbed. If you have a rest at the same time don't be tempted to sleep with your baby on a sofa or couch – put him in a basket (or his pram).

Bedtime

When it comes to going to bed it is important to set up a routine that becomes calming and comforting and becomes intrinsically linked with sleep. Ideally this should be followed from around six weeks old.

Babies initially sleep for the majority of the time – up to 18 hours a day in the first few weeks. This tends to be slightly less (around 15 hours) by three months. But remember, your breastfed baby will probably not sleep more than three to four hours at a time as your breast milk is absorbed more readily than formula milk (which tends to keep baby feeling full for much longer).

The first two to three weeks are likely to be fairly unpredictable and it is difficult to maintain a routine at this stage. However, you should start trying to set up a routine between two and three months after birth, in order to settle your baby ready for sleep. Be consistent in this routine in order to convey a positive message promoting sleep. At this stage it is worth trying to start putting your baby down awake, although sleepy, in order that he can learn to fall asleep without having to be 'fed to sleep'. If your baby always falls asleep on the breast, then when he wakes or stirs in the night (as invariably he will at some point) he will not be able to get himself back to sleep without going back on the breast.

Q. How do I start to set a bedtime routine?

It is worthwhile starting to set up a routine for bed when your baby is between two and three months old. For example, you may be able to incorporate bath time followed by a quiet but interesting time which will become associated with going to sleep. The consistency of this routine becomes predictable and familiar to your baby, who will be more relaxed when he knows what is happening next.

What you do in this bedtime routine is ultimately your choice, but don't start playing any games that may get baby too excited; if you start the routine downstairs, maybe playing a game, or in the bathroom, finish it in the bedroom.

Here are some suggestions for a bedtime routine:

- You could start with a bath, which can give your baby a chance to use up some energy, kicking his legs and splashing. You could take the bath together, with baby in the bath with you, or he could go in with your partner, who may enjoy having this special time with baby too. This could be an ideal opportunity for your partner to be involved and could also give you a bit of free time to relax.

- Some parents make a routine out of saying goodnight to all those around, including favourite teddy!

- You could then have cuddles and read a story before breastfeeding and then put him into his cot before reading him a story.

- Many babies settle well if you play some soft music or a lullaby tape when you leave them.

- You could sit in his room for a short while, reading or singing to him before leaving him with some music playing to let him settle to sleep.

Q. My baby tends to fall asleep at the breast and then wakes as I put him down.

If he falls asleep at the breast do be prepared for him to stir, if only momentarily, when you first put him into his basket/cot/bed. If you can, finish feeding him so he is on the arm with which it is easier for you to lay him down. If this doesn't happen naturally, simply move him on to that arm when he has finished feeding. Then, if he does stir when you lay him down, keep your arms around him – don't pick him up again, just rest against him, so he can feel secure. As he grows more accustomed to this you can gradually withdraw, using just your hand on his body, then sitting near the cot.

Do ensure that your baby has a good feed at this time – he will not go to sleep if he is still hungry. If he is seems unsettled initially, leave him for 5 or 10 minutes to see if he will settle, but if he still seems unsettled after this it may be worth checking that he is not still hungry, in which case he may need to go back on the breast once more. This can be tricky, because you don't want him always to fall asleep on the breast as this can cause problems when he wakes and finds no breast. However, don't be tempted to drop the routine or take him back downstairs as this will just reinforce his behaviour. Be consistent with this routine and your baby will respond.

Settling baby to sleep – Charlotte's experience

Charlotte was breastfeeding her son, Harry, with few problems, except that Harry loved being on the breast. At bedtime, following his bath, Charlotte usually read Harry a story and sat quietly with him, talking. She would then give him his 'bedtime feed'. Harry attached properly and would suck and feed well. As a result he would generally fall asleep, at which point Charlotte would attempt to put him in his cot. Halfway through this procedure Harry would often wake, crying, and Charlotte would then repeat the process of breastfeeding Harry to sleep and try all over again. Sometimes this would also happen following a 'night-time' feed.

This can sometimes be a problem because, as your baby feels so snug and secure, when he is then put into a 'cold' cot he may stir and possibly even wake. The best way to overcome this will depend on the age/size of your baby and what he is sleeping in. As Harry was now sleeping in a cot I suggested it would be beneficial to adjust the height of the mattress. This is very useful providing your baby is not yet able to sit up unaided. Many cots now have the ability to allow the mattress to be raised higher, so it is not necessary to bend too far into the cot in order to put baby down. Then by dropping the cot-side, this allowed Charlotte to stay close to Harry once he was actually lying on the mattress. I advised her to keep close to him whilst putting him into the cot, even to keep her hands and arms around him for a little while, once he was on the mattress, in order to let him drift off again. Before leaving Harry she could then raise the cot-side back into position.

If your baby is still quite young, you could try putting him into a Moses basket or carrycot, first, and then place that into the cot. When you first put him into the basket he may stir — just rock the basket gently and this might help to soothe him back to sleep.

Charlotte generally sat in a chair for their bedtime routine, so I asked her to look at how she moved from that position into a standing position, as this can in itself cause some disturbance. She would need to ease herself towards the edge of the chair in order to then be able to stand up in one smooth easy movement. I also suggested that she tried to ensure she ended the feed holding Harry on the side which made it easier for her to be able to put him into his cot.

I advised Charlotte to keep the bedtime routine calm, with low lighting and perhaps some music playing quietly in the background which can again help lull baby off to sleep.

These changes helped to relieve some of the problems Charlotte faced in trying to get Harry to sleep and subsequently she became practised in these so it was less of an ordeal each evening.

Q. Should baby have his own bedroom?

Every parent and professional will have their own view on this. Personally I believe that when putting your baby down to sleep at night it may be best to keep him in the same room as you for the first six months at least. This is often, practically, a very sensible idea; you are going to be getting up to feed at least once, often more, during the night. This way, you don't have to walk too far to get baby; and mostly this *will* be you – few partners want active involvement during the night feeds, especially after the initial novelty wears off.

During the bedtime feeding routine, keep the lights dim; if you have a small plug-in nightlight you may find this is sufficient to be able to see. Talk quietly and soothingly to your baby and don't be tempted to 'play' – concentrate on breastfeeding and then put him back in his cot. You need to make baby realize that there is a difference between night and day and that this is not time for playing.

Babies should be put in their cot, on their back with their feet at the bottom of the cot. You should not use duvets or pillows for children under the age of one year old, nor is there any need to have cot bumpers around the sides of the cot. They may look pretty but they can increase the temperature around your baby, which can lead to him becoming overheated, so they are not advisable.

Safe bed sharing

The safest place for your baby to sleep overnight is in a cot close to your bed. If your baby is born preterm, is ill or has a high temperature it is probably better not to bed share.

However, you may wish to take your baby into your bed for breastfeeding as this can be far more relaxing for you, rather than sitting in a chair feeling as if no one else is awake or exists at that time of night. If you do this there are certain precautions to take, as you may feel quite sleepy while breastfeeding:

- Neither you nor your partner should have been drinking, smoking or have taken any substances that mean you are very sleepy and unlikely to be able to respond to your baby; this includes any medications you have been prescribed by your doctor.
- There should be no gap between the bed, headboard, mattress or wall where your baby could roll and get stuck.
- The mattress should be firm, not sagging and not a waterbed.
- Light coverings rather than a duvet on the bed will help prevent your baby overheating.
- Similarly, do not overdress your baby, or have the room too warm.
- If another child is sharing the bed, you should be between the child and your breastfeeding baby.

Baby's temperature

Q. How warm should the room be?

You will probably notice that your bedroom feels a lot cooler than the ward or room when you were in hospital, but less clothing and blankets are used in hospital because it is so warm.

When you come home you need to ensure that the room(s) you are using are warm but not too hot – around 16 to 20 degrees is about right. It can be a little less than this and it won't hurt baby.

Your baby cannot really control his temperature until he is two to three months old, so be aware that you will need to check on him. You should be aware of how warm he feels and adjust his clothing and bedding as needed. For the first four to five weeks a good guide is that your baby needs one more layer of clothes than you do to be comfortable.

Obviously in winter you may find that the rooms are cooler, especially the bedrooms overnight when any heating may not be on. This may result in baby waking if he gets cold, but do not use an electric blanket in the cot. Check the TOG values of clothing and bedding and try to aim for a total TOG rating of between 10 and 12. This should ensure your baby is warm enough but not over-wrapped. There is no need to use a hat or mittens indoors; only if the room were quite cold would mitts really be necessary. To check how warm baby is, feel his body – around his back, between the shoulders – not his hands and feet which are often more chilly.

TOG values of clothing and bedding

Vest		0.2
Babygro		1
Jumper		2
Cardigan		2
Trousers		2
Disposable nappy		2 (this will be less if it is wet)
Sleepsuit		4
Sheet		0.2
Blanket	– old	1.5
	– new	2
Quilt		9

If you swaddle your baby (i.e. wrap your baby up within a blanket) this trebles the TOG value of that item of bedding.

Night noise

Q. My partner snores. Will this disturb my baby?

Babies do settle when in the same room as you and your partner. Don't worry too much about whether your partner's (or your own) snoring will wake the baby – these sounds are often reassuring to your baby.

You may find that you are aware of your baby's little noises during the night. Remember that this is a good thing. If you are roused as he starts to wake for a feed he will not be upset by the time you have reached him. These preparatory noises also alert your body so that letdown happens more readily once you do start to feed your baby. As already mentioned, there is some debate about whether you should have your baby in your room or put him in his own room. Many people are keen to 'put baby in his own room' as soon as possible (often on arrival home from hospital) and decorate the nursery especially for him.

This doesn't happen in many other cultures; the baby usually stays with his parents in their room, sometimes for the whole of the first year.

You may find friends and family starting to tell you 'not to spoil him' and that you should put him in his own room. However, it is so much easier to have your baby in your room, especially when you are breastfeeding several times a night. Neither of you are completely wide-awake and this helps promote the comforting feeling; it can then be easier to get baby back to sleep afterwards. If you adopt this approach it can be helpful as baby is comforted by your presence and the movement of you/your partner can act as triggers to your baby, encouraging him to adopt a similar breathing pattern to you. In the first few weeks many new mothers want to check on their baby's breathing during the night; if he is in the same room as you this is much easier. Be prepared, though, to hear a less regular breathing pattern in your baby than in another adult. Often the more irregular breathing and 'murmurings' are when your baby is in a 'dreaming' sleep and you don't need to worry about this. He is likely to have a more regular breathing pattern during a deeper quiet sleep period.

Night feeding

Q. Is it really necessary to breastfeed during the night?

Remember that the milk production hormone, prolactin, works overtime during the night, so any night-time feeds really do help boost your milk supply.

It is hoped that you will have fed your baby soon after delivery and then as frequently as he wants to, remembering that the more often he feeds the more often prolactin (the milk-producing hormone) is released and the greater the supply of milk produced. Your baby may be quite sleepy in the first 24 hours following birth, but ideally he should take about three or four feeds in his first 24 hours. However, following this he is then more likely to want to feed every two to three hours, especially when your milk has 'come in', from around day 3 or 4. You should then let your baby feed as often as he wants and for as long as he wants to, providing he is correctly positioned and attached properly – breastfeeding rather than 'nipple sucking'.

So, during these first weeks it is important not to miss any feeds, and although you may be relieved if your baby sleeps straight through the night, this can affect your milk supply. The night feed is associated with much higher prolactin levels, which means your milk supply is stimulated even more, so try to cope with these night feeds during these early days.

Often by about six to eight weeks your baby will begin to sleep through the night, perhaps feeding at around 10 or 11 p.m. and then waking again at around 5 or 6 a.m. If this happens when your baby is much younger, you may wake up with a very full feeling in your breasts and the lack of regular feeding can affect your milk supply. However, some babies may take until around five or six months of age to start sleeping through. This doesn't mean you are doing anything wrong, just that all babies are individual; but attempting to keep to some form of routine can be helpful, and it is best to establish this earlier rather than later.

Q. So, if my baby does sleep through the night earlier than this should I wake him?

No, there is no need to wake him. If your baby doesn't wake during the night then he is probably ready to sleep through and will get all the milk he needs during the day. Remember, this may change again when he has a growth spurt, so he may actually start to wake again.

Oxytocin, the 'letdown' hormone, also helps to induce relaxation in both you and baby, which will ensure that both of you are more ready to sleep following a breastfeed. It is also thought to help with 'bonding'.

Maintaining your lactation

Q. What about growth spurts?

Remember 'baby-led' feeding – your baby should feed when he needs to and this will ensure that your milk production meets demand. There will be times when your baby undergoes a growth spurt and this will usually involve him increasing his demand. Just respond to this and feed more frequently and your milk supply will quite quickly adjust to this increased requirement.

Once your breastfeeding has become established it is usual to expect to feed six to eight times in a 24-hour period. If your baby is feeding less than this in the first couple of weeks you may have less success at breastfeeding. There is no need to give your baby any extra fluids as all he needs is contained in your breast milk. Sometimes it may be suggested that you give extra water if the weather is hot, but again this is not necessary; instead, you may find that your baby wakes for a 'short' feed in between his normal feeds due to being thirsty. Just respond to this, so if you are feeling warm and need to drink more, then it is just as likely that your baby does too.

Q. If my baby seems constipated, should I give him extra water?

Occasionally someone may suggest giving your baby a drink of extra water if he seems constipated. Constipation in a breastfed baby is very unlikely so this is not necessary. However, if your baby is being given formula milk or has started solids it may be more likely.

So, if you are giving artificial milk to your baby you may want to consider the following:

- Make sure that you are making up the formula correctly, adding the right amount of water.
- You may be able to help stimulate bowel movements by helping your baby to relax, putting him a warm bath and then gently carrying out a tummy massage.
- You may also try putting a little cream/Vaseline just around his bottom; don't be tempted to put anything inside his anus (bottom). Occasionally you may hear suggestions to insert a thermometer inside the anus to help stimulate the bowel. This is really to be avoided as it may cause damage to the delicate tissues inside the anus.
- You could give extra water to your bottle-fed baby, but this is likely to reduce the amount of milk he takes.
- Fruit juice can be given to infants over the age of six months, but it should be diluted, one to ten parts, with cooled boiled water.

Q. How many calories should I eat when I am breastfeeding?

You should ensure that you have an adequate diet; you don't need to eat for two, but you should have a balanced diet. Eat and drink regularly to satisfy your own hunger and thirst, rather than because you think you should consume a certain number of calories. However, your diet should be nourishing and healthy, not all chips, crisps and chocolates. What you eat is providing the nourishment for your baby; and you will need the energy to provide your breast milk. Don't worry about eating a little more than usual as you will use up those calories in feeding, but don't overdo it. Once your lactation is more established, just be guided by how hungry you are feeling.

Q. Are there any foods I shouldn't eat?

Although there is often some worry that certain foods, such as spicy foods, garlic or citrus foods, may upset your baby, there is no need to avoid any particular foods. On the whole, eat your normal diet, but not an excess of anything, and observe any reaction in your baby. You may find that if you do eat a large amount of a particular foodstuff your baby is more windy the following day, but if this is not causing him any distress there is no need for you to avoid that food. It takes between about two and six hours for a foodstuff to 'come through' in your milk, so you could try to determine whether a particular food may have had any effect on your baby.

If you do notice your baby is a bit unsettled after you have eaten something, leave it out of your diet for a few weeks, then retry it; if it has the same effect it may be wise to avoid it until baby is a little older. However, if milk or dairy foods seem to be causing a problem then speak to your GP or midwife/health visitor for some advice. Avoiding dairy foods is a major undertaking and involves eliminating a very important food group from the diet which should be done only with medical advice in order to avoid problems later.

Often babies who have been breastfed do seem more willing to try different tastes when the time comes for weaning, probably because they have become used to different tastes that come though in the milk.

Remember that everything you eat ultimately goes to your baby via your breast milk, so do be aware of the amounts of substances such as caffeine (in tea, coffee, some soft drinks, chocolate and some medicines), nicotine (this can also reduce the milk supply), artificial sweeteners and in particular alcohol you are consuming. It is certainly better to avoid smoking altogether and may also be best to avoid alcohol while feeding.

Q. I thought breastfed babies had fewer dirty nappies, but my baby seems to dirty his nappy every time I change or feed him.

For some babies this is quite normal and as long as this is his usual pattern then that is exactly what it is – normal, for him. In some ways this is a good sign; it shows his digestive system is working well and that he is getting enough milk.

Babies who have fewer dirty and wet nappies tend not to be getting sufficient milk. So in the first few weeks don't worry about this.

Any stool should be soft, often mustard coloured and maybe a little watery, but if it is very liquid or smelly this could be diarrhoea which may need to be checked out by your doctor. However, as your baby grows you may find the number of dirty nappies per day does settle down.

Weight gain in your baby

Q. Why has my baby lost weight since he was born?

All babies will lose a certain amount of weight in the first few days after birth; this is usually around 8 per cent of their birth weight. Most babies will then regain this weight by 10 to 14 days of age. Part of this weight 'loss' is because your baby passes his first stool – meconium, a thick greenish-black tar-like substance – within the first 24 hours.

Colostrum within your milk acts as a laxative, so this helps your baby to get rid of this meconium. If your baby doesn't seem to be regaining his weight you need to speak to your midwife.

Make sure you are feeding your baby as often as he needs and make sure he is latched on to your breast properly. If, after the first week, he seems to be a little sleepy during feeds without taking very much, try talking to him while you are feeding, or tickling his toes to ensure he proceeds with the business of breastfeeding. If he is sleepy, look at the section on jaundice in Chapter 07 as this can sometimes be responsible for sleepy babies who are not too keen on feeding.

Keep a check on the number of wet and dirty nappies your baby has – there should be at least six wet nappies a day by around day 5. The stool your baby passes will also change, going from the black tarry substance, through a greenish colour (at around day 3 or 4), to a loose or soft 'mustard-yellow' stool when your milk has 'come in'. The stool of the breastfed infant is not particularly offensive; it has a rather characteristic smell which is slightly sweet and cheesy.

As long as you notice that your baby is going through these changes in his stool then you can be reassured that your milk supply is adequate. If, however, he is still passing meconium at day 4 or 5 this could indicate that he is not receiving sufficient breast milk for some reason.

Q. When I take my baby to clinic I worry he is not gaining the right amount of weight.

On average babies gain around six ounces per week, although this does vary with the individual and whether or not you are exclusively breastfeeding. Also, if your baby is born prematurely, or is a twin or multiple, this is less accurate. Most babies will tend to double their weight by six months, but again the information upon which this is based was taken from primarily formula-fed children.

Breastfed babies tend to gain weight quickly in the first few weeks; this then slows and by the time they are ready for solids they are often gaining less than many of the growth charts suggest they should. However, if your baby is otherwise happy, alert and active then this is nothing to worry about.

The growth charts can be useful but often lead to anxiety, especially for you. Try to remember that a 'one-off' weight is less useful as it needs to be looked at within the context of other weighings and the age of your baby. If you and your partner are small, then your baby is more likely to be small too – this is quite normal. Any weight must be seen in relation to others, so if there is a gradual slowing down of your baby's growth, or if he seems to have stopped gaining weight over a longer period, this is more likely to need investigation. See Chapter 07 for more about weight loss.

How to increase your milk supply

Putting your baby to the breast more frequently is the best way to increase your supply, so if your baby seems to be hungrier – perhaps going through a growth spurt (this is quite common at around three to four months) – this may be something to think about. Do check that your baby is positioned correctly and is suckling effectively.

Certain medicines, for example the contraceptive pill (especially the combined pill), some antihistamines and ephedrine-based medicines can reduce your supply. So if you are taking, or planning to take, any medicines you may need to discuss this first with your doctor or pharmacist.

If you have been giving your baby any extra bottles (of formula milk or even water) this could have affected the amount of milk 'demanded' from your baby and therefore reduced the amount of milk you are producing. In order to increase your milk production you should cut out any additional feeds and concentrate on increasing the number of times you breastfeed your baby or express your breast milk.

If your baby uses a dummy this can also reduce his demand and so reduce the number of times he feeds, which in turn will affect your milk supply. Your baby may have been comforted by the dummy, which stopped him feeling the need for the breastfeed and the milk he required. So it is best to avoid using a dummy if possible.

Also, in between feeds you can massage your breasts and express your breast milk, which will encourage greater milk production. If your baby is in a neonatal unit (special care) this massage and expression can also be helpful.

Breast massage

Q. Why should I massage my breasts?

Breast massage has been shown to increase the amount of prolactin released, which in turn increases the amount of milk you produce. It should be done gently and alongside expressing your breast milk.

- First, wash your hands.
- Then sit somewhere comfortable with some degree of privacy. If you have something with you to remind you of your baby, such as a photograph or a blanket that smells of him which you can have close, this can be helpful in initiating your 'letdown'.
- You can also use warm flannels around the breast tissue to help stimulate the flow of milk.
- Using your first two fingers, gently rotate them in a circular motion over your breast tissue.
- Massage from the outer part of your breast, moving down towards the nipple. Continue this all around your breast.
- You can also hold your hand in a fist and roll the fingers gently downwards from the outer part towards the nipple area.

- This can be followed by stroking your breasts from the outside towards the nipple area.
- You can gently roll your nipple between your thumb and first finger to help stimulate your hormonal responses.

You should attempt to carry out this massage for around five minutes prior to expressing the milk; you can repeat it half-way through expressing if you feel the milk supply is dwindling.

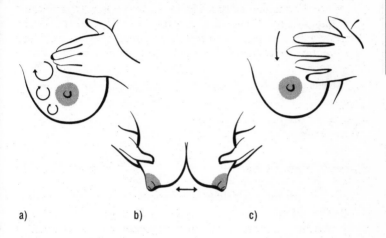

a)   b)   c)

figure 5.1 breast massage

Expressing your milk

If you need to express milk for your baby it is advisable to massage your breasts first, as described above. When you have spent a short time massaging your breasts you can then start to express your milk.

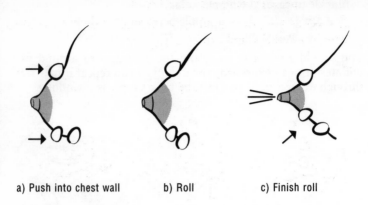

a) Push into chest wall   b) Roll   c) Finish roll

figure 5.2 expression of breast milk

- Place your hand, with your first two fingers and thumb forming a 'C' shape, around your breast.
- The best position for fingers is around 2–3 cm from the base of your nipple.
- If you feel around the area, you will notice there is a difference in the texture of the tissue under your fingers – you should place your fingers and thumb over the area where you feel this difference.
- Push your fingers/thumb in towards your chest wall (Figure 5.2a) and then 'roll' them back towards the nipple in a press-and-release movement (Figure 5.2b).
- This movement should be directed backwards towards the chest wall, rather than a squeezing movement of the thumb and fingers.
- Try not to drag or slide your fingers over the breast tissue as this can result in friction, causing damage. You may find this is more likely if your breasts or hands are wet, so try to keep them as dry as you can.
- Then move your 'C'-shaped hand around the breast tissue so that you express all around the breast, not just focusing on one particular area.
- Lean forward, hold a wide-necked, sterile container in your other hand and squeeze the drops of milk into this.

- Continue to express your breast in this way; if the milk flow slows then change to the other breast.

The whole process should take no longer than 20 minutes, including massage and expressing.

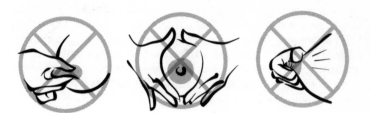

a) Do not squeeze   b) Do not slide   c) Do not pull

figure 5.3 what not to do when hand expressing your breast milk

Using a pump

Q. Do I have to use my hands to express milk?

Not necessarily. You can, of course, use a pump to express your milk; however, it is not really necessary. Prolactin response is actually better when breast milk is hand-expressed than when using a breast pump. But if you prefer there are a number of pump varieties to choose from – manual or motor. You may be able to obtain a hand-operated pump on free prescription.

Manual pumps include those that are operated using a trigger-style mechanism, those with a cylinder and those using a rubber bulb mechanism. These varieties are less expensive but may be limited in the amount of milk they can collect before they needing emptying. Motor-operated pumps may be battery or electrically operated. Electric pumps are usually found in hospital and can be quite expensive, although it may be possible to borrow one of these, perhaps from your local maternity unit or a local National Childbirth Trust branch. With these pumps it is usually possible to undergo 'double-pumping' (both sides at the same time), which can be more efficient.

If you do decide to use a pump then it will also be necessary to sterilize all its components, which can be difficult with some of the parts. It is certainly worthwhile to try hand expression initially. There is no cost involved in this method as no special equipment is required, just a wide-necked container and clean hands, and it is far more gentle than using a pump. The use of hand expression is far more like the natural suckling action of a baby. The suction strength of the electric pumps can often be too strong; this can vary with the size of the pump. With some types of pump it is possible to adjust this suction strength.

Using and storing expressed milk

You can give the expressed breast milk via a supplemental feeding system (see Chapter 08), which can allow you to increase the amount your baby takes at a feed; this can be useful if you are concerned about your baby's weight gain. You could give this breast milk to your baby fresh, or store it for later use.

Q. How can I store my expressed breast milk?

You can keep your breast milk in the fridge or freeze it. If you are going to store milk in the fridge or freezer you should cool it quickly first, by standing it in cold water.

There are lots of different guidelines given for how long you can store expressed beast milk, but the current recommendations are given here:

- Expressed breast milk stored in the fridge should be kept in the coldest part – not in the door – at 4°C or below for three to five days.
- If you wish to freeze milk, you can use sterile plastic bags, or small plastic containers – leave at least 1 cm of space at the top of the container. Label the container with the date you expressed the milk.
- You can store expressed milk in a fridge-freezer for up to three months, or a deep freezer for six to 12 months.
- Defrost expressed milk as quickly as possible when you wish to use it, but not in a microwave. Defrosting expressed milk in a microwave can destroy some of the nutrients, so it is better to remove it several hours before you need it and leave it to thaw in the fridge.

- Alternatively, if you need it quickly, hold the container under a running tap, starting with cool water and gradually increasing the temperature of the water; or stand it in warm water for 20 minutes.
- Once thawed, this milk can then be kept in the fridge for up to 12 hours. However, any milk not used within this time must be thrown out – do not refreeze it.

Returning to work

You may intend, or need, to return to work following the birth of your baby – this does not mean you can't breastfeed, or that you need to give up breastfeeding. However, it does mean that you need to be organized and to think ahead. How you cope with the demands of breastfeeding may depend how old your baby is when you return to work. You may be very lucky and have a whole year off with your new baby, or at least several months; on the other hand you may be back at work within five to six weeks.

There are several options you could think about:

- When looking for childcare it may be possible to find somewhere near to your place of work; perhaps your employer has a work-based nursery. This would give you the possibility of being near to your baby, so you can feed him before you leave for work, visit during the day when another feed is due and feed him again on collection. However, this may not be possible for many women, so you will need to consider other possibilities.
- It may be possible to return to work part time or to job-share for a period of time, so you only work two and a half days per week.
- Perhaps you could extend your period of maternity leave.
- Alternatively, consider the possibility of returning to work and expressing your milk while separated from your baby. This milk can then be given to your baby by your child carer. You will need to discuss this with your child carer to ensure they understand your wishes and know how to reheat your expressed breast milk.

  Q. Does my employer have any obligations to help me continue to breastfeed?

  Your employer is not legally required to have a breastfeeding policy but you are protected, by law, if you wish to continue to breastfeed on your return to work. You need to find out if your place of employment has a breastfeeding policy, which will ensure your employer is legally obliged to help you to continue to feed. This may include the possibility of letting you work more flexible hours for a while, or allowing you a 'breastfeeding' break.

You need to inform your employer in writing, on your return to work, that you wish to continue to breastfeed. Your employer should then conduct an assessment to assist you. You should be provided with a clean, quiet and private area to use while you express your milk – this should not be the toilet – and somewhere to store your milk.

However, if you work for a small company you may find that there are no guidelines on breastfeeding/expressing, which can make it more difficult for you to discuss your needs with your employer.

There is further information regarding your rights as a breastfeeding mother to be found on the Health and Safety Executive (HSE) and NHS websites. These addresses can be found in the 'Taking it further' section at the back of the book.

If you decide to express milk while you are at work, you will need to decide how you are going to express your milk. You can buy a pump to express your milk, but this has to be cleaned and sterilized before use so may actually be more difficult from a practical point of view. You could hand express, which means that there is no need for any other equipment. This option is sometimes easier as you may not be able to wash and sterilize the different parts of the pump following its use. You can use cool bags to transport your milk home.

It is probably a good idea to practise hand expression before you go back to work so you become fairly accomplished and are able to do it easily. It is also useful to start expressing before your actual return to work as you can start freezing your milk in order to build up a supply to leave for your child carer.

When back at work, you may find you feel engorged (or even experience leaking) at certain times during the day and if so, this indicates when would be a good time to express your milk. You will discover which are the best times are for you. However, don't worry if you do not experience this engorgement – it does not necessarily mean you won't have enough milk. Your body might just be adapting better to the changes.

When expressing your breast milk, change sides when the flow slows down, unlike when actually feeding your baby. This changeover seems to help stimulate your letdown. On average you can expect your baby to need about $2^1/_2$ ounces per pound of his body weight, per 24 hours. So if your baby weighs 10 lbs, he will require about 25 oz of milk in 24 hours. This rough guide is based on formula-fed babies and so you can expect your breastfed baby to differ from this slightly, some days taking more or less than this and the intake may not be distributed evenly throughout the day.

Going back to work – Mandy's story

Mandy had been breastfeeding her son, Tom, since birth and had to return to work after six months. She worked full time and needed to continue to do so on her return. She could not take any part-time work, and if she failed to return to work would have had to repay her maternity leave pay, which she could not afford to do. Although there was no workplace nursery available, she was lucky enough to find a place at a nursery very close to her place of work.

I had demonstrated to Mandy how to hand express her breast milk as, although there was a private area she could use, it may have been difficult to be able to wash and clean any equipment used to express her milk at work. She had practised at home for a few weeks prior to returning to work and found that she was quite successful with hand expression.

Following my advice, Mandy fed Tom prior to setting off for work. Expressed breast milk from the previous day was given to the nursery staff to give Tom during the day. Mandy was very productive with her breast milk and supplied sufficient milk for Tom's needs. Some of this milk was used to mix with some solids; the remainder was used as extra milk feeds during the day. The milk was given to Tom from a beaker with a slow flow spout.

Mandy expressed her breast milk around lunchtime, collecting it in a couple of wide-necked bottles. This milk was then kept in a cool bag until Mandy got home and transferred it to her fridge. Once at home, she offered Tom another breastfeed, then later, a meal of some solids. She breastfed Tom again before he went to sleep. Tom settled well into this routine and continued to breastfeed as more solids were introduced. Mandy finally stopped breastfeeding completely at 18 months, when Tom was happy to sleep without his final breastfeed.

Had the nursery been closer to Mandy's workplace, it may have been possible for her to visit during the day and breastfeed Tom, which would have been particularly useful if she had returned to work prior to the introduction of solids. However, Mandy was very happy with the result, particularly as she had been quite keen to avoid giving Tom any formula milk, as there was a strong history of allergies within the family.

Adjusting to your return to work

How your body adjusts to your return to work and maintaining breastfeeding will depend on you, at what stage you return to work and how many hours you work. For some mothers there is no problem, their breasts adjust and they can express sufficient milk to leave for their baby when they not there, while others may find they have less milk over time. However, remember that it will depend upon the age of your baby when you return to work – he may not require as much milk as previously, so you may find you have sufficient milk to supply his needs. There are fewer problems in maintaining your lactation if you return after your baby is four months old as your lactation is generally well established by this point.

When you are with your baby in the evenings, at weekends and so on, return to your usual feeding routine and put your baby to your breast.

If you work part time there will be other times when you can continue feeding your baby, which will help maintain your milk supply. Many women find that their body does adapt and they are able to continue to breastfeed their baby; this will also depend upon the age of your baby and how long you have been breastfeeding. It is not a good idea to try to return to work within the first couple of weeks following delivery while trying to establish your lactation. This is also to be discouraged for your own benefit as you need to rest and recover – you will tire more easily as you are unlikely to be getting sufficient rest in those early weeks.

Feeding your baby expressed milk

The expressed breast milk can be given to your baby mixed in with food if he has started solids, via a cup or beaker or via a bottle.

If you intend your baby to be fed your expressed breast milk from a cup or bottle it is a good idea to try to introduce this prior to your return to work. This will reassure you that this method will work for your baby, although do remember, if you are trying to feed your baby with a cup or bottle, he can smell you, so he may be more interested in trying to nuzzle up and find the breast. This is usually less of a problem when someone else is trying to feed your baby with expressed milk.

There are some cups/beakers available that have a variable flow 'teat' which are very useful for breastfed babies needing a cup. These allow you to adjust the flow of milk being given so your baby learns to swallow smaller amounts; young babies tend not to be able to drink directly from a cup initially so this is an ideal 'in-between' product to help your baby cope with a cup.

You may not wish to use a bottle if you are worried about your baby adapting to the different sucking action required when using a bottle. Some babies will adapt to this, while others won't and so refuse a bottle. If you have tried to introduce feeding your baby expressed milk from a bottle prior to your return to work and had problems, don't worry – many breastfed babies are reluctant to take milk from a bottle, especially if it is their mother who is holding the bottle. Let your partner, or better still, your child carer give your baby this milk in the bottle; or try to introduce a cup. This is often more successful as your baby does not have to adapt his sucking action while taking the milk.

Summary

- If possible, start expressing your milk several weeks before you return to work in order to build up a store of expressed breast milk.
- Practise the method of expression so you feel comfortable carrying this out.
- Remember to discuss this with your employer and find out if there is a breastfeeding policy within your workplace.
- Try giving your baby expressed breast milk, introducing a cup or bottle. This may be achieved more effectively by someone else, as your baby will expect a breastfeed from you.
- Discuss your wishes with your child carer and ensure they are able to store and reheat your breast milk correctly.
- You will need to purchase containers in which to collect your milk and a cool-bag for transporting it home. You may wish to buy a pump, although hand expression is more convenient and economical as it requires no equipment and no sterilizing. Sterilization equipment will be required if you are using cups or bottles and your baby is under one year old.

Breastfeeding your adoptive baby

If you have adopted your baby, you may wish for the chance to breastfeed. This is still possible, even if you have never had a baby or breastfed before. However, the amount of milk you can produce will depend upon how old your baby is when you adopt him. In most cases you will still have to supplement your baby with formula milk, but putting your baby to the breast and allowing him to suckle will stimulate prolactin release. The amount of prolactin will influence milk production, so the more your baby can suckle at your breast the more breast milk you will produce. The length of time needed to produce breast milk will vary with each individual, but sometimes milk will be produced within just a few days. Even though you have not been pregnant, this will still have the same effect.

Q. Will I have enough breast milk for my adoptive baby?

It is unlikely that you will be able to exclusively breastfeed your adoptive baby as you will probably not produce sufficient breast milk to be able to fully feed him. You will start to produce breast milk in response to your baby's needs, but it will take several weeks to produce the volume of milk needed to fully feed your baby. However, by this time your baby will have grown more and so his milk requirements will have increased further, so there will still be a shortfall in the demand and supply. The younger the baby, the more successful you are likely to be; those under three months old are more successful in being able to exclusively breastfeed than older babies.

In order to start to breastfeed your adoptive baby, you will need to use a supplemental nursing system (sometimes called a 'Lactaid'). This will allow you to give your baby a formula feed while he is suckling at your breast, so at the same time stimulating prolactin and milk production. The advice relating to attachment and positioning will be the same for your adoptive baby as for other babies, but further information about using a supplementer can be found in Chapter 08.

Feeding your preterm baby

The difficulty in delivering your baby before your due date is that there is a greater chance that he will be smaller, less well developed and less resilient. He may well need some medical help or interventions shortly after birth, and may need to be transferred to a special care or neonatal unit, which may interfere with the initiation of breastfeeding.

If possible, try to have some skin-to-skin time with your baby before he is transferred for any care; however, if this is not possible don't worry, you will probably be able to do this within the neonatal unit where your baby is cared for, just ask the staff looking after him. If you are separated from your baby before attempting to breastfeed, it is very important that you try to express your milk sooner rather than later. The earlier you start expressing, the better. Breast milk is particularly important for your preterm baby as it is specifically suited to his needs. There are a number of reasons why your preterm infant benefits from your breast milk, including helping to improve his growth and development.

Benefits of feeding your preterm baby breast milk

- It will lead to improved growth as breast milk is made to suit your baby at whatever gestation he is born.
- Development of the brain and visual development are enhanced.
- It helps to protect against a rare but serious condition of the bowel (necrotising enterocolitis), which mainly affects preterm infants.
- Preterm breast milk has higher levels of a number of ingredients, such as protein, fatty acids and energy.
- The right nutrients are in a concentrated form, which suits the preterm infant who has a small stomach and an underdeveloped digestive system that takes longer to digest any foodstuff.
- There are also higher levels of immune factors in preterm breast milk that help give an increased level of protection.

Q. Will I be able to breastfeed my preterm baby?

If your baby is born very early it may be difficult for him to breastfeed as his reflexes may not be developed enough and he is likely to tire easily. In this case you can express your breast milk so that this can be fed to him.

It is important that you try to express your breast milk every three to four hours, ideally six to eight times in a 24-hour period (including at least once during the night), saving the milk in a sterile container. The neonatal staff will then be able to give it to your baby. This may be via a feeding tube initially, depending upon how early your baby has been born.

As your baby grows and develops the method of feeding will change; if your baby has been fed by tube, cup feeding will usually follow next, which helps your baby to develop the skills needed for breastfeeding.

Don't worry if in the first few days you only express a few drops of milk – this is still of vital importance. The colostrum and early milk will contain valuable nutrients and antibodies to help your baby's immunity, and the amount will increase if you continue to express regularly.

As soon as you can you should put your baby to your breast, even if this is only for part of the feed, and then continue to express your breasts to ensure your supply is maintained.

The paediatrician (baby doctor) and neonatal staff will help you to continue breastfeeding and expressing. You may be advised (for some of the time) to try 'double-pumping'. This is achieved using an electric pump to express both breasts at the same time. This has been shown to be helpful to obtain maximum amounts of breast milk. Usually a pump will be available within the neonatal unit for when you visit your baby, although you may need to hire a pump for use at home if this is advised. When expressing your milk, whether by hand or pump, it is useful if you can be near your baby at this time, or have a photograph of him and an item of his clothing with you; this helps your oxytocin response and letdown release.

When your baby is ready you will be able to put him directly on your breast, gradually building up the time he spends there; so you should continue to express throughout the time your baby is on the neonatal unit as it will help you maintain your supply. During this period you will usually be encouraged to give your baby skin-to-skin contact as this helps him to be aware of your smell and touch. Your partner can also have skin-to-skin contact with your baby from time to time to help them bond.

Coping with twins or more

Having twins or a multiple birth does not mean you cannot breastfeed, although you may need more help initially, especially when trying to latch them on simultaneously. Your body will be able to meet the demands of both babies, as the increased demand will result in an increased supply. However, you may find you do need more rest as it can be more tiring feeding more than one baby. You need to look after yourself and make sure you have a healthy balanced diet; concentrate on looking after yourself and your new babies until you feel breastfeeding is going well.

One at a time or both together?

It is possible to feed twins either simultaneously or individually, i.e. one at a time. Feeding one baby at a time allows you to focus on that baby specifically and can be easier when trying to ensure correct positioning and attachment; however, this may mean that you have less time in between feeds.

Feeding both babies together can be easier as they get older and you become more confident; and it is possible that (like 'double-pumping') simultaneous feeding provides greater stimulation and helps in the early days to start and build up the supply of your breast milk.

It is usually best to feed your twins in much the same way as a single baby, so if you are just feeding one of the twins, you should swap the baby from one breast to the other if he still wants more after being on the first breast.

If you are feeding your twins simultaneously, it can be a good idea to ensure one baby does not always feed from the same breast, as one baby may have a stronger suck than the other and so could stimulate that side more. However, you may find that your babies show a preference for one particular side and it might be that keeping to one breast ensures that the milk is more suited to that baby and means he gets sufficient hind milk (milk produced towards the end of the feed).

So, for the first few days it may be helpful to feed your babies individually in order to ensure they are positioned correctly, progressing to simultaneous feeding as you become more experienced.

Of course, it will also depend upon how often your babies wake for feeding, although if one or both are small you may be advised to wake them for feeds. It is also more likely that your babies will be delivered prematurely if you have twins, which again can mean they are likely to be smaller and may have problems in sucking; see the previous section on preterm infants.

Most mothers who have multiple babies do have ample milk to feed both babies, and many continue to breastfeed for over 12 months.

Feeding positions for twins

Q. What is the best position to use to feed my twins?

You may need to consider the positioning of your babies if you do wish to feed them simultaneously. The easiest hold to use is the 'rugby-ball' hold, although you will need to be sitting on a settee rather than a single chair and use pillows to support the babies. A U-shaped or triangular pillow can be helpful in assisting you to hold your babies in this position. Initially you may need to help one baby latch on by supporting your breast from underneath. This is when it is easier if you have someone to help, who can then hand you the other baby so you can repeat the process of latching him on to the other breast. There is no need to swap them over partway through the feed – just allow them to come off the breast spontaneously. Then wind them if necessary. It is very important to ensure that both babies are positioned and attached correctly in order for them to obtain sufficient milk and gain weight.

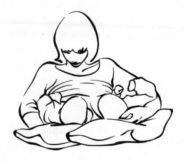

figure 5.4 feeding twins using the 'rugby/football' hold, sometimes called the 'double-clutch' hold

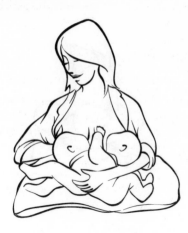

figure 5.5 feeding twins using a 'cross-over' hold

Another option is the 'cross-over' hold. However, this may not be tolerated by the baby who is lying under his twin, especially as they grow older. Use a pillow/cushion under your babies to bring them up towards your breasts.

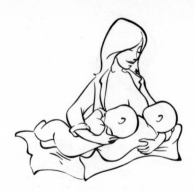

figure 5.6 feeding twins using a mixed or parallel hold

If you use a mixed or parallel hold, both babies are lying in the same direction, supported with pillows/cushions.

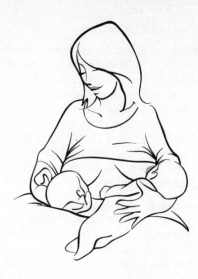

figure 5.7 feeding twins using a combination hold – cradle/clutch hold

Using a combination hold allows one baby to be held under your arm in a rugby-ball hold while the other baby is held in a cradle hold.

It is important to choose the position that you find most comfortable and easy. Whichever position this is, ensure you are not holding either of the babies' heads at the back as this will prevent them from extending their head should they wish to. Make sure you are sitting up straight, not leaning forward into your baby, otherwise you will get very tired. When feeding twins you may sometimes feel the need to give one of your babies a bottle; where possible it is better to use expressed breast milk for this. If you express following feeding, this can allow you to build up a store, which could be used when you feel the need for a 'relief bottle'.

Teeth

Q. Can I still breastfeed if my baby has teeth? Will it hurt?

Very rarely are babies born with teeth; however, at some time, usually between four and eight months old, your baby will start teething. It is hoped that you will still be breastfeeding at this time, but you may be a little worried about continuing to feed when your baby has developed some teeth. The first teeth to erupt are usually the two lower front incisors, but remember that if your baby is attached correctly at the breast, the tongue covers the lower gums (and therefore the teeth), so these teeth should cause no problem while he is latched on.

Although the lower teeth will generally be protected by your baby's tongue when he is feeding, occasionally as the feed comes towards an end, your baby may fall asleep and may 'nip' you unintentionally. Or, if he is distracted during the feed (if someone comes into the room or there is a noise that interests him) he may turn towards it and take the nipple with him, biting it at the same time. This usually results in a rather immediate response from you, in the form of a scream or shout; the result of this is a rather startled baby. Often this is enough of a shock to your baby to ensure he does not repeat the offence. Your response may be so sudden as to frighten your baby and you may need to calm him down. You should try and stay calm, say a very firm 'No', look directly at your baby and stop the feed. He will then understand this is not a game. If he is biting, put your little finger in the corner of his mouth between his gums – don't try and pull him off as this may cause more damage.

Biting is generally not intentional, but some babies may repeat the action to see if it produces the same effect in you. If this happens you must show your displeasure and remove him from the breast at that time; he will associate these two actions and normally this will stop any repeat biting. Sometimes your baby may bite in an attempt to ease the discomfort in his gums, so a cooled teether may be useful for him to chew on. Alternatively, you could use a teething gel, or chamomilla, to rub on to his gums. Don't apply it to the tongue as some gels can numb the tongue, which can then make it difficult for your baby to latch on to the breast.

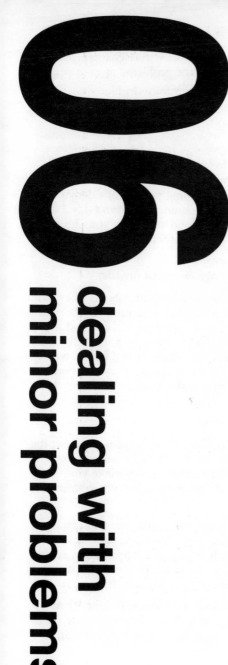

06

dealing with minor problems

In this chapter you will learn:
- about breast engorgement
- about sore or cracked nipples
- about mastitis and blocked ducts
- about thrush infection
- about inverted nipples.

Most mothers will experience a problem at some point during the time they are breastfeeding. If you are lucky enough not to, that's brilliant, but for those less lucky, this chapter provides some advice to help you through the problems or even prevent the problem occurring in the first place.

Engorgement

Q. What is engorgement?

Engorgement is when your milk comes in faster than your baby can take it away, so exceeding your baby's demand for a while. It tends to occur quite suddenly, around day 3 or 4, as there is also an increased blood supply to your breast at this time, ready to supply the nutrients necessary to make your milk.

Q. How will I know if I have engorged breasts?

You will know you have engorged breasts as they will suddenly feel very tender, swollen and lumpy. The extra blood supply to your breasts makes them feel full and heavy and you may feel warmer than normal. It is usual for both breasts to be affected and the whole of the breast will be involved. If they have swollen to such an extent that the nipples are flattened this may make it difficult for your baby to latch on well.

Q. What causes engorgement?

There are generally two reasons for engorgement. First, the amount of blood going to your breasts increases to supply the breast with the necessary ingredients to make your milk. It is around this time colostrum changes into transitional milk.

Second, the hormone prolactin starts to stimulate the secretory cells in your breast to produce a greater amount of milk. Prolactin is present all through your pregnancy, getting ready for breastfeeding your baby, but it only really starts to work after you have delivered the afterbirth (placenta).

Perhaps engorgement shouldn't be considered as a problem – it is your body coping with the new demands being made on it. But, if you are experiencing engorgement, it will certainly feel like a problem to you.

Preventing breast engorgement

- Feed regularly – every couple of hours.
- Feed when your baby wants to – be 'baby-led'.
- Ensure that your baby is latched on correctly.
- If feeds are consistently very long, check that your baby's positioning at the breast is correct.
- Avoid the use of supplementary bottles of formula milk as this can disrupt the supply and demand mechanism.
- Allow baby to come off one breast on his own, before offering the second breast.
- Don't drop the night-time feed, especially in the early days – be prepared to keep it going until your baby is at least six weeks old.

Q. My milk came in today and my breasts feel as if they are swollen to twice the size they were. They are hard and painful. Why is this?

Lots of mothers feel like this around the third or fourth day and often decide not to even try breastfeeding because they are worried about painful engorgement. But engorgement will happen regardless of whether you intend to breastfeed. This is because the hormone levels in your body have risen ready to feed your baby and will dwindle over the first week, so engorgement will still be felt. However, this engorgement is temporary and will usually subside within 24 to 48 hours.

During the first few weeks of breastfeeding your body is learning to supply just the right amount of milk for your baby's needs (supply and demand), and to start with there will be some over-production while this mechanism adjusts.

In the beginning your baby will probably be feeding every couple of hours, which will help to stimulate your milk supply. So when your milk 'comes in', it is produced faster than your baby can consume it. This is often more noticeable if this is your first baby. Mothers breastfeeding their second or third baby may not have a problem with engorgement. This is probably because they feel more confident with breastfeeding and have established a pattern from the start.

The engorgement will resolve itself within a couple of days but in the meantime it is important to keep feeding regularly – every two to three hours. You may notice your baby becomes quite 'fussy' around the time the milk comes in, and wants to breastfeed even more often, almost as if he can't get enough of it. Do feed whenever your baby wants to, but make sure he is attached and positioned correctly – if he isn't he may not be able to remove the milk as effectively, which will lead to further engorgement.

If you don't intend to breastfeed, don't try to express the breast milk to get rid of it and make yourself feel more comfortable, as your body will think your baby is simply trying to increase the supply and so will make more milk to supply those needs.

Q. My breasts are so tense and swollen it is very difficult to latch my baby on. What can I do?

Engorgement can result in the nipple becoming flattened and this makes it more difficult for your baby to latch on. If so, express a little milk (use your hands or a pump) prior to feeding your baby, relieving the engorgement slightly and allowing your baby to attach. Don't express too much as this may encourage more production. Warm flannels applied to your breasts before you attempt to breastfeed will also help to soften your breasts and encourage the 'letdown' reflex.

Q. Is there anything I can do to make my breasts feel more comfortable?

If you are suffering from breast engorgement there are several thing you can do to relieve the discomfort. These are discussed below.

• Make sure you continue to breastfeed during the night. Of course, this is the time when no one really wants to be awake, but the night-time feed gives the best prolactin (milk-producing hormone) response, so your milk production will be better too. Think of this night-time feeding as a temporary phase and just enjoy this special time with your baby. But make sure you catch up with your rest during the day – when your baby naps, you should too. Don't be tempted to try and get all your little jobs done while he is asleep. Usually the night-time feeds will come to a natural end as your baby settles into a pattern. You may be lucky in that this might happen at around six weeks of age, although some babies continue until later, perhaps three months. Very occasionally a baby never seems to want to sleep through the night and still demands his feeds – this may need looking at differently as it could be that he has got into a habit, rather than actually needing a feed due to hunger.

- When your baby goes through a growth spurt you may notice that he starts to wake for a feed earlier and this is a good time to increase the number of times you feed for a few days while your body adjusts again.
- Make sure baby is positioned correctly and is properly 'latched on'. If your baby regularly takes a long time to complete his breastfeed (more than an hour) it is most likely that he is not latched on properly so is not feeding well.
- Use warm flannels before breastfeeding to soften your breasts and help your 'letdown'. Soak a flannel in warm (not hot) water and then put them on your breasts around the areola area (the darker area around the nipple). Or you could sit in the bath or stand in the shower and let warm water spray onto your breasts, which can give you some relief too.
- Express a little breast milk before feeding to help your baby 'latch on'. When you have used the warm flannels, gently massage your breasts to help the letdown and then you can gently express a little milk, just enough to soften the area around the nipple and areola so your baby can latch on more easily. Don't be tempted to overdo this as this will be seen as a signal by your body to supply more milk.
- If your breasts still feel quite full after your baby has fed well, don't express more milk from them as this will lead to an increased production for next time.
- Change baby's feeding position. It can help to make sure all the ducts in your breast are emptied if your baby adopts different positions from one feed to the next. So try to use a different position, perhaps move from a cradle hold to a rugby-ball hold at different breastfeeds.
- A supportive bra is a must. Make sure the straps are wide and don't cut into your shoulders. Wear this even at night, but make sure it is not too tight, as any pressure from this will be painful when your breasts are engorged.
- It can help to put cooled 'gel' packs (available from chemists) inside your bra. This helps to ease the inflammation. Use these after you have finished a breastfeed.
- Another remedy is the application of chilled cabbage leaves to the breasts. This has been suggested for use in severe engorgement and some women find this is helpful. The cabbage leaf should be refrigerated before application to the breast, with a hole cut in the leaf to allow the nipple to go

through. The leaves should be left in place for about 20 minutes, until they have warmed to body temperature.

• Finally, a simple analgesic can be taken if the discomfort is severe. Remember that engorgement is temporary and really is a good sign as it demonstrates that your body is working to meet your baby's needs.

Summary – coping with breast engorgement

• Use warm flannels or showers before breastfeeding.
• Offer frequent unrestricted feeds.
• Use cold compresses or gel packs in bra after feeding.
• Wear supportive bras.
• Apply chilled cabbage leaves (Savoy are best) to the breast area, inside your bra, between feeds. Leave them in place until they have reached body temperature.

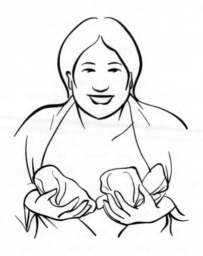

figure 6.1 apply cabbage leaves to your breasts to ease engorgement

Q. So if I am feeding my second baby and don't experience any engorgement, does this mean I will have less milk?

No, many second and third time breastfeeding mothers don't necessarily experience engorgement. This is probably because you are more experienced in putting your baby to the breast and feel more confident, so have probably been breastfeeding your baby regularly from the start. It may be that your breasts are more able to adjust to the supply and demand with subsequent babies.

Severe engorgement

Severe engorgement is when the breasts feel rock hard and are swollen. This can occur if engorgement is not dealt with successfully. It is due to lymph congestion and only tends to happen if engorgement has not been managed properly at the beginning, so it is important to continue to let your baby breastfeed when your breasts are engorged in order to allow your body to regulate the supply and demand of milk.

Severe engorgement can be very painful and you may feel unwell, hot and shivery. This can affect your breastfeeding, as the milk sacs (alveoli) in the breast become so distended that they are unable to contract and expel milk, and so the secretory cells in the breast are flattened and are unable to produce milk.

Another problem is that there is a substance in your breast milk that inhibits milk production while there is already milk in your breasts. So, if your baby does not breastfeed well and take sufficient milk due to engorgement, this substance will inhibit any further milk production because your body thinks your baby has had enough. This will ultimately affect your lactation, as your baby will not be able to get enough milk to meet his needs. The measures suggested above may help and at times a mild analgesic may be necessary.

If you are having problems with engorgement, either speak to your midwife or breastfeeding counsellor, or contact an advisor from the National Childbirth Trust or La Leche League (see 'Taking it further' for more details on these organizations).

Sore nipples

Q. I am fair skinned and have red hair. Am I more likely to suffer from sore nipples? Should I start to prepare my nipples for feeding?

Not at all. It used to be said that certain women were more likely to experience sore nipples and that certain practices could prevent them. None of this is true.

Sore nipples are a problem best prevented! They are usually caused by poor positioning and attachment of your baby during breastfeeding – pain is nature's way of telling you something is wrong. Breastfeeding should *not* be painful. Certainly in the first few days it can be a strange sensation when baby clamps his jaws around your breast tissue and, especially if he has a strong suck, it can initially make you catch your breath; but once he is on the breast and sucking this sensation should go. You should feel able to relax your shoulders, uncurl your toes and not feel any pain.

Try to think of this initial discomfort as nipple sensitivity, after all, they have not been exposed to this particular stimulation before so may initially be quite tender, but not painful. Any sensitivity should disappear once baby is attached and suckling well. If you are still feeling pain then something is not right – you need to check the positioning and attachment of baby at the breast. This can be difficult to do yourself and you may need to ask your midwife to help you. Sometimes it is only a matter of an adjustment of a couple of millimetres, but this can make all the difference.

Even if you have breastfed before, this doesn't mean you won't experience some difficulty this time. This may be because your breasts are slightly lower than with your first baby. You may try and put your new baby to your breast in exactly the same way as before, which may not be quite right this time round. Read the suggestions for how to get baby to the breast in Chapter 03.

If your baby does not get the nipple into his mouth correctly or does not have enough of the surrounding breast tissue in his mouth it is easy to damage the nipple, resulting in soreness. Try changing the position you feed in and ask your midwife or partner to look at how the baby is attached.

If you are feeling soreness or pain when baby is feeding, take him off by breaking the seal between his mouth and your breast with your little finger and bring him back to the breast again. You may need to do this several times until he learns how wide he needs to open his mouth.

Q. I have heard about nipple shields. Could I use one of these to breastfeed with?

Nipple shields (often shaped like floppy 'Mexican hats') are not a good idea. There may be less pain initially but this is not solving the problem. The main cause of sore nipples is poor positioning and attachment, so if your baby goes to the breast in the same way using a nipple shield, he will still be latched on incorrectly. This means that the nipple is likely to be damaged further. The problem of getting baby latched on correctly must be tackled to resolve this issue. If you do use a nipple shield you may find some blood around your nipple; you may even see a small amount of blood coming out of your baby's mouth, as the nipple is being damaged. This won't harm your baby but it is a sign that the problem causing the soreness is not being dealt with.

Sore nipples and nipple shields – Helen's story

Helen was trying to breastfeed her second child, Sarah. She had previously breastfed her son, four years earlier, with few problems. However, she contacted me as she had been experiencing very sore nipples, in particular on the left side where the nipple was starting to crack. She had mentioned it to her midwife, who had suggested applying some 'spirit' to her nipple, but warned this would make them sting! Instead, Helen went to her local chemist and was advised to try using nipple shields. Although she had been told these were not usually recommended, she was desperate and so purchased a pair and went home to try to breastfeed again.

On using the nipple shields she found little difference in the amount of pain she was experiencing and when she looked down at her daughter feeding, noticed a small trickle of blood oozing from her mouth. She was absolutely aghast. When she looked at her nipple it was now bleeding. I visited her following her frantic phone call telling me this sad tale.

I asked Helen to put Sarah back on the breast, both sides, and watched her technique. It was obviously very painful for Helen, especially on the nipple that was now cracked. From my perspective the answer was obvious. She was using a 'cradle-hold' on the left side and a 'rugby-ball' hold on the right side. This was part of the problem. Helen was putting Sarah to the breast the same way (i.e. at the same angle) for both sides, just as she had when she fed her older son. The 'angle-of-dangle' of her breasts and nipples had changed since her previous feeding experience and her nipples actually pointed out at slightly different angles. I adjusted Sarah's feeding position and suggested that Helen used a 'rugby-ball' hold on both sides, which seemed to improve the position of the 'latch'. Although she still felt sore initially, once Sarah was actually feeding, this improved and there was no longer pain throughout.

I advised Helen not to continue to use the nipple shields as, rather than improving the state of her nipples, they were contributing to the problem as her nipple was hitting the inside of the shields and causing further damage.

Within the next couple of days Helen noticed a gradual improvement; she continued to manage to feed on both sides. However, if she had not been able to bear the pain when feeding on the one side, she could have fed from the other side and expressed the milk from the more painful side for a couple of feeds. This would have allowed the cracked nipple time to recover, especially if a little expressed breast milk were rubbed onto the nipple and left there between feeds.

Q. Are there any creams I can use?

You will find a number of creams, ointments and sprays available to treat sore nipples, but for some women they may actually make the problem worse if they are sensitive to the ingredients. Creams and ointments will not resolve the problem unless the issue of positioning is tackled and dealt with.

To ease sore nipples you could express a small amount of breast milk and apply this around the nipple. Don't wash your breasts and nipples with soap and try to keep them dry in between feeds. When you can, try to let the air get to your nipples as this will help stop them getting 'soggy'. This is fine if you are at home alone, but not very convenient if friends drop by or you wish to go out! For these times try putting a small plastic tea strainer (with the handle cut off) into your bra cup, so your nipple is covered by the strainer and not touching your bra. This will allow them to air-dry and not sit soaking in wet breast pads.

Sore nipples can lead on to engorgement as you are not removing the milk effectively, so you do need to solve this problem. Some babies are very eager when they first go to the breast, and suck very strongly, so try feeding from the side which is least sore first. Then, when baby has quenched his initial hunger or thirst, you can take him off that breast by gently breaking the suction with your little finger (don't just pull or you will cause more damage) and put him on the other side.

Some women find they prefer to feed from the side which is most sore first as they then can relax into the feed, knowing the worst bit is over. You may wish to try this, especially if your baby likes to play with the nipple towards the end of the feed. This is more likely to lead to sore nipples.

If you really think you are doing everything you can and still feeling pain, do contact someone for help and advice. This could be your midwife, as she is probably still visiting you at this time, or a support group such as La Leche League, National Childbirth Trust or other local group. Details of these groups can be found in 'Taking it further'.

Do try to keep feeding, however painful this may be for you. If you stop breastfeeding you are likely to that find that your breasts continue to fill and become engorged. If you really cannot face putting your baby to the breast, or on one particular side, express your breast milk for a couple of feeds. Do this gently, by hand if you can as this is more gentle than using a pump. Details in how to do this are given in Chapter 05.

Summary – dealing with sore nipples

- Prevention is far better than cure – try to ensure that your baby is attached and positioned correctly from the start.
- Do not accept that breastfeeding has to be painful – it should not be. Pain indicates that something is not quite right.
- Check your baby's position and attachment.
- Try adopting another position for feeding – if you usually feed in the cradle hold, try the rugby-ball hold, or lie down. You may find using a different position for each side works better.
- Creams/lotions and sprays are not usually very helpful. Instead, express a little breast milk after the feed and gently apply it around your nipple.
- Don't let your nipples become soggy – wet breast pads are not a good idea. Try leaving them exposed to the air, either when you are having a lie down or are alone in the house.
- Use a cotton bra rather one made of synthetic material.
- An adapted tea strainer inserted into your bra cup can protect your nipple and allow some air around it to keep it dry.

Cracked nipples

This may be the result of sore nipples that have not been dealt with successfully. Again, prevention is the best treatment here. The same advice will apply as has been given for sore nipples, and as long as you do not find it too painful you can continue to feed.

So, make sure that your baby is attached correctly with a wide-open mouth and has the areola in his mouth, not just the nipple. Try to expose your nipples to the air after feeds and keep them dry, not next to soggy breast pads. Leave a little breast milk on the nipples after the feed as this can help to heal them.

Cracked nipples may be made worse by dryness and friction, so if this is the case then a non-irritating cream may help, just as lubricating dry or cracked lips are relieved by lip-salve. The use of a thick cream such as highly purified lanolin (not an oily product like Vaseline), unless you are sensitive to this product, may help with the healing process. However, the root of the problem, i.e. ineffective attachment, must be dealt with.

Sore and cracked nipples are sometimes associated with a thrush (candida) infection. This will be discussed later.

Mastitis

Mastitis is an inflammation of the breast. You may notice a red, swollen area on the breast, which will usually be painful. Normally only one breast will be affected, and usually this will be confined to a small section (one or two lobes) of that breast. Mastitis can occur if engorgement is not relieved, or it may be the result of a blocked duct.

Signs of mastitis

- There will be a reddened area on part of the breast – usually this is the upper, outer part, nearer the armpit. This will probably be a wedge-shaped area as often only one lobe is affected.
- The breast will feel hot to the touch.
- You may feel generally unwell, with flu-like symptoms, a high temperature, shivering and aching.
- The breast area will be painful to the touch.

A blocked duct will stop your milk flow and may be felt as a small lump (like a bead) around the areola and can occur if your baby is not correctly attached and so does not 'empty' part of the breast effectively. It is due to an inflammation rather than something physically obstructing the ducts.

This may happen when your baby's feeding pattern changes, for example if he misses a feed or sleeps through the night. It may be caused by pressure, perhaps from your bra being too tight, or you may have pressed your finger over part of your breast in an attempt to give baby's nose space (this is not necessary).

Q. What should I do if I have mastitis?

Mastitis is usually self-limiting, although occasionally it can require antibiotics. However, the first measures you take must include putting baby to the breast as frequently as possible, and putting your baby to the affected breast first. Placing your hand over the red, inflamed area while baby is breastfeeding on that side can help to encourage drainage of the area. You may feel tired and feverish with this and you can take some paracetamol or ibuprofen to relieve these symptoms.

The use of refrigerated cabbage leaves has been helpful for a lot of women. Or you could use a small bag of frozen peas applied to the area (especially after a feed) to help relieve the symptoms. This, together with regular feeding and emptying of the breast, is often all that is required.

If the condition persists, and you continue to feel worse and despite trying the measures suggested above you see no improvement within 12 to 24 hours, then you should see your doctor. At this point antibiotics may be needed if you are found to have infective mastitis, but these can often be avoided.

It is not usually necessary to stop breastfeeding while taking most antibiotics; your doctor should be able to prescribe those that do not affect your breast milk. However, you may notice a slight reduction in your milk supply following an episode of mastitis. Increasing the frequency of feeds can overcome this reduction in supply. Don't be tempted to reduce your feeding at this time, even though you may feel unwell and low in yourself – it is likely to risk making your symptoms worse or lead to a reoccurrence. Make sure you have sufficient rest and drink plenty of fluids.

If you do need to take antibiotics there is a small chance that these can pass through your breast milk, which can occasionally lead to your baby suffering temporarily with diarrhoea and being more at risk of thrush. However, it is still better to continue to breastfeed than to introduce artificial milk at this stage.

Q. Should I stop breastfeeding if I have mastitis?

No, don't stop feeding – feed as often as baby wants to, and if your breast still feels lumpy following a feed, you could also express to try to clear the blockage. Look at the position you normally feed your baby in, and perhaps think of changing this. Sometimes it can be more comfortable feeding your baby in the 'rugby-ball' hold as it can encourage drainage of the ducts while not putting pressure on your breast.

Some other suggestions for helping to relieve mastitis:

- Make sure your bra is not too tight or restrictive and that it is the right size; avoid under-wired bras while you are breastfeeding.
- You can help the milk flow by applying warm flannels or running warm water over your breasts before feeding, and you may wish to express a little before feeding to soften the area first.
- You could also use breast massage to help relieve mastitis – see the section in Chapter 05 on breast massage. Massage gently above the tender area; you can do this while baby is breastfeeding to help to clear the blockage.

Breast abscesses

Mastitis or a blocked duct that has not fully resolved can lead to a breast abscess (where there is a collection of pus), but this is not a common condition. You will need to see your doctor for this and often the abscess will need to be drained. You may also be prescribed antibiotics. You can continue to breastfeed from the unaffected side, but check with your doctor whether it is advisable to feed from the affected side. If you are advised not to feed from that side, express the breast milk from that side and throw it away. This should only be necessary for two to three days. Do not suddenly stop breastfeeding as this may mean a worsening of the problem and you may find yourself with mastitis in both breasts.

Q. How would I know I have a breast abscess?

You may have developed a breast abscess if you can feel a small lump, often with some redness, in your breast. You may see some pus in the milk or leaking from your nipple. You will generally feel unwell, as with mastitis, and you may find the area painful due to the pressure in the breast from the abscess.

Summary – breast abscesses

- These can occur as a result of an unresolved blocked duct or mastitis.
- You may notice a reddened area and a lump in your breast.
- There may be some pus discharge from your nipple or pus in the milk.
- You will feel unwell and may experience pain in the breast.
- This needs medical attention – often antibiotics are given and the abscess may be drained (either lanced or aspirated).
- Do not stop feeding suddenly.
- You can feed on the unaffected side. If you are advised not to feed on the affected side, express the milk from that breast for a couple of days.

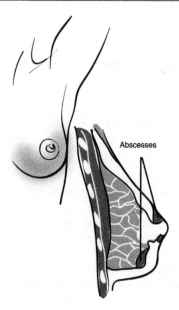

figure 6.2 position of breast abscess

Thrush (candida infection)

Thrush is a fungal infection caused by an organism called *Candida albicans*. This is a yeast organism that lives normally around your mouth and vaginal area without any problems. You may be familiar with thrush as you may have experienced an infection yourself. Some women suffer with thrush during pregnancy as a result of the effects on the vaginal area of hormonal changes.

Candida thrives on carbohydrates and so the sugar (lactose) in your breast milk is ideal to help it grow and reproduce. If you have taken antibiotics for any reason, this can allow the yeast organisms to multiply because the 'friendly bacteria' that normally maintain the candida balance may be killed by the antibiotics along with the infection.

Thrush can affect your breast and so pass on to your baby and affect his mouth (this is known as oral thrush). This can then continue to pass back and forth between you and your baby. Thrush may not be immediately diagnosed as it can start as sore nipples and be thought to be due to poor positioning and attachment. Thrush can cause soreness long after the initial feeding period and so may arise after a period of otherwise problem-free feeding.

Q. My breasts are very pink and sore and I have a deep pain in my breast. What can this be?

This could be a sign that you have a thrush infection of your breast.

Symptoms of thrush

- You may notice that your nipples are very sore and not improving. No amount of attention to positioning seems to help, as this is not the cause of the problem.
- Sometimes your nipples may feel burning, itchy and flaky as well as sore.
- You may also experience a deep pain within your breasts, which will continue throughout the feed and often in between feeds too.
- You may also experience intense shooting pains within your breast during or after feeding. Sometimes this can indicate that thrush has entered the ducts within your breast.

- You will notice that your nipple area is very red and shiny, and often itchy. Very occasionally you may see white spots around the nipple area.

If you recognize any of these symptoms, look in your baby's mouth – if he also has thrush, his mouth will be red and you may see white spots in his mouth. These could be mistaken for specks of milk, but if you try to wipe one away with your clean finger or a cotton bud it will look raw and sore underneath. Your baby may not be keen to feed and may seem irritable, probably a result of his sore mouth.

You may also notice that your baby has a red bottom (nappy rash) which could be a result of thrush.

How to recognize thrush (candida)

- You may have very sore nipples; they will be very red and shiny.
- Your nipple area may also be hot and itchy.
- You may experience deep breast pain within your breast, during or between feeds, and sometimes sharp shooting pains either during or after a feed.
- Occasionally you may notice white spots around your nipple area.
- Often baby will be affected as well, so look for signs of redness/soreness or white spots in his mouth.
- Your baby may also have a sore, red nappy area.
- Baby may be irritable and less keen to feed if he has oral thrush as his mouth will be sore.

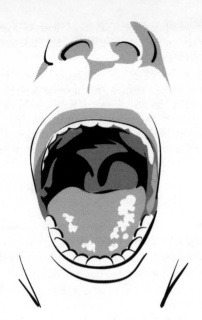

figure 6.3 oral thrush in baby's mouth

What might help?

The following may help with the prevention and treatment of thrush:

- Try to keep your nipples dry, as the yeast responsible likes moist warm conditions in which to grow.
- Wash your breasts and nipples but avoid soap – plain water is better.
- When you can, let your nipples 'air dry'.
- Try eating natural live yoghurt which contains bacteria that can help fight against thrush; this will reduce your susceptibility to thrush. It is also very soothing if you apply live yoghurt on and around your nipples.
- Make sure you wash your hands and take care with personal hygiene.
- Change disposable breast pads with every feed or wash non-disposable breast pads regularly.
- If you are wearing cotton bras, these can also be washed at high temperatures to eliminate the organisms.

This condition will need medical treatment as soon as possible. It will not clear up without it. You can purchase antifungal creams over the counter from pharmacists, but be sure to ask for a preparation suitable for treating the nipple area. It will probably be necessary to treat your baby as well – your doctor can prescribe a liquid suspension for the mouth and/or cream for the nappy area. It is usually necessary to treat both you and your baby at the same time in order to ensure there is no chance of cross-infection. If the infection is in the ducts it may be necessary for you to take an oral course, such as Nystatin, which your doctor can prescribe.

It is possible to have recurrences, so to avoid this pay particular attention to personal hygiene, and any other family members should be treated at the same time. It is also vital to remember to adequately sterilize, or dispose of, anything that comes into contact with your baby's mouth – such as teethers or dummies if you have been using these. This organism is very difficult to get rid of as it has heat-resistant spores, so be scrupulous about sterilizing.

Although there may be times when it is necessary to use antibiotics during your pregnancy or following delivery, try to avoid using them if you can, as they can predispose you to a thrush infection. Eating live yoghurt can help reduce your likelihood of infection, or you could take acidophilus tablets, which are available from health food shops or chemists.

If you do start treatment, be sure to continue with it for the prescribed period; remember, the more severe the infection the longer it may take for the treatments to work and for you to be pain free again. Don't be tempted to give up – if the problem does not resolve, see your doctor as a different antifungal remedy may be required.

Inverted nipples

Only a very small number of women will have inverted nipples.

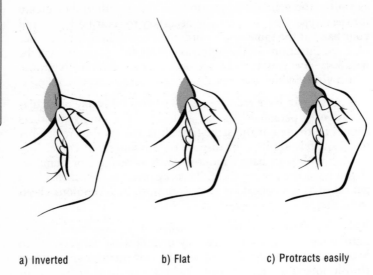

a) Inverted   b) Flat   c) Protracts easily

figure 6.4 types of inverted nipples

There are two types of 'inverted nipples' – flat or truly inverted. If you think you may have inverted nipples you can try 'the pinch test' during pregnancy. Gently pinch the area around the nipple, about an inch from the base, with your thumb and first finger. The nipple may protrude, which is a good sign; however, if your nipple does not protrude then it is probably 'flat'. If it tends to fold inwards (retracts) and disappears then it is truly inverted. This may change during pregnancy as the hormones can cause the nipple to protrude. Each breast may be different, so you may find only one side has an inverted or flat nipple. However, as your baby should attach to the areola tissue (the darker area around the nipple), not just the nipple itself, this should not mean you cannot breastfeed.

It is very important that your baby is positioned and attached correctly in order to ensure he has a mouthful of breast tissue to form a 'teat', which will enable him to obtain your breast milk. Encourage your baby to latch on, getting a 'mouthful' of breast tissue. This may be more difficult if your breast is engorged, so do try to feed regularly.

Q. I've been told I have inverted nipples. Are there any exercises to correct this?

There have been a number of exercises suggested and devices promoted which supposedly help to correct inverted nipples. But actually none of these have been proven to be of any help. In some cases there has been evidence that some of these treatments could actually cause nipple damage and really should be avoided. Breastfeeding with truly inverted nipples can be very challenging and will require skilled help and a lot of patience.

Often, as the baby grows, it does become easier to breastfeed from inverted nipples. Also, if only one breast has an inverted nipple it is possible to breastfeed quite successfully using just one breast.

Now let's move on and look at health concerns you may have about your baby.

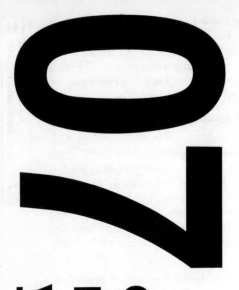

07 concerns you may have about your baby

In this chapter you will learn:
- how to recognize if your baby is not gaining sufficient weight
- how to cope with your unsettled baby
- how to tell the difference between vomiting and reflux
- how to tell if your baby is constipated
- how to tell if your baby is milk intolerant
- about jaundice in babies
- about tongue-tie.

This chapter is intended to cover some of the concerns or worries you may have with your baby and give you some tips on how to deal with them.

Weight loss/poor weight gain

Your baby will be weighed following his birth, and over the next three to four days you can expect him to lose between 8 and 10 per cent of his birth weight. This weight loss is quite normal and expected, and you should then see your baby start to gain weight, regaining his birth weight by 10 to 14 days after his birth. Part of this weight loss is due to the changes that happen following delivery – the first stool your baby passes (meconium, the first dark stool) – and will be influenced by how your baby has fed and the amount of colostrum he has been able to take.

Remember that in those first few days your baby may be weighed on several different sets of scales, which could all give slightly different readings. Also, your baby's weight can alter depending on the amount of clothing he is wearing when he is weighed – it is best to be consistent in the amount of clothing he is wearing each time.

Your baby will obviously be weighed at birth, but your midwife may then not weigh him again until day 4 and then once more in the first week. Sometimes your baby may not be weighed until day 7, depending on your midwife. After the first ten days he may be weighed less frequently, especially if he has regained his birth weight. Don't become too focused on your baby's weight – if he is feeding well, sleeping, having several wet nappies each day, passing mustard-yellow soft stools and seems contented, alert and responsive when awake, there is probably little to worry about.

Signs that your baby is healthy

- He feeds well at least six to eight times per day (depending on his age).
- He has several wet nappies each day (which do not smell) – up to six after the first week.
- He is passing soft mustard-yellow stools after the fourth day when your milk has 'come in'.
- He is alert and looking around.
- He sleeps well.
- He has good skin colour – not pale or grey.
- He seems happy and contented.

Q. When do babies have growth spurts?

Once your milk has come in you will find that your baby starts to gain weight quite quickly. Be aware of growth spurts; these typically occur at around two weeks, six weeks, 12 weeks and six months. Around these times you may need to increase the frequency of feeds in order for your milk supply to meet this increased demand. Most babies double their weight within the first four to six months; however, be wary of values used on some growth charts.

Some of the charts used to interpret the weight gain of your breastfed baby were designed over 50 years ago and were not necessarily related to breastfed infants in their early months of life. So, you may find that your baby gains more weight than expected from the chart. Once feeding is well established, a breastfed infant will gain weight more rapidly than may initially be expected. This growth rate does tend to slow down once weaning begins and solids are introduced, i.e. for the second part of the first year. This is a normal pattern for your breastfed infant.

Q. My baby doesn't seem to be gaining weight. What can I do?

If your baby doesn't seem to be gaining weight and you are becoming concerned then increase the frequency of breastfeeds.

Let baby suckle for as long as he wants, ensuring first that he is positioned correctly. If feeds regularly last longer than an hour, and your baby is sucking throughout, not falling asleep, then you need to check that he is attached and positioned correctly. Remember that if you supplement your breast milk with a bottle (even if this is only water) you will reduce the amount of breast milk your baby demands and your supply will similarly reduce.

What could cause your milk supply to decrease?

- Taking the contraceptive pill.
- Pregnancy.
- Trying to extend the time between feeds.
- If you introduce bottles of formula milk; the more often he has a bottle the greater the impact on your milk supply.
- If you try to do too much.
- Certain medicines can affect your milk supply.

Q. My baby is feeding well but not gaining weight. What is happening?

Very occasionally when your baby is several weeks old, he may be feeding frequently but not gaining weight. He may also be passing large amounts of urine and having frequent, loose stools that are green and frothy. He may be miserable and appear colicky. Your breasts may feel persistently full and leak often. This can be linked to an over-production of milk (often only temporarily), of which the baby is taking mostly the low-fat 'fore' milk. So, although he is getting large volumes of milk, it is too low in fat and calories to assist good weight gain.

If you are over-producing milk and your baby is getting mainly fore milk, the best way to deal with this is to express some milk prior to putting your baby on the breast. This will remove some of the fore milk, so when your baby feeds he will receive more 'hind' milk, which is higher in fat. This will mean that he takes in more calories, so he will then be more satisfied and have a longer gap between feeds.

You can also try to reduce this problem by demand-feeding your baby in the early days, whenever he wants. You can also collect milk from the other breast if it is leaking, while you feed from the other side – then store this or donate it to a 'milk bank' if there is one locally. Some maternity units have milk banks where donated breast milk is collected from local breastfeeding mothers. There is a national organization that organizes donated breast milk supplies. Contact details can be found in 'Taking it further'. This milk is then used, following pasteurization, to feed small, ill and preterm babies.

If your baby generally feeds from both breasts at each feed it can be useful to offer only one breast at each feed (alternating which one is offered) for 24 hours. This will usually allow the milk supply to be more equal to demand and then your normal feeding can continue. See which of these works for you – usually you should see results within only a couple of days so you could adjust your feeding pattern to suit you and baby.

For a short time, until your supply settles to meet baby's requirements, you may wish to use plastic-backed breast pads when going out, to protect your clothes (and your dignity!). Don't use them all the time though, as this will keep the nipple area too warm and moist and can lead to thrush and sore nipples.

Coping with too much milk

- Express a little milk prior to putting baby to the breast, but don't overdo this.

- Instead of feeding from both sides every time, feed from one breast at one feed, and the other breast at the next. This will ensure that your baby is getting the hind milk, which is higher in calories, not just low-calorie fore milk.

- It can take up to a couple of months for your milk supply to become balanced against the needs of your baby.

An unsettled baby

If your baby seems constantly to be demanding attention and not settling after feeds this can be very draining for you and you may begin to wonder if you are doing something wrong.

During your first few weeks of being a new mother you are on a steep learning curve trying to understand what your baby needs – it is all very new, so don't be too hard on yourself. In the early days your baby will usually cry for a reason: hunger, wind, wet/dirty nappy, or from being tired; the problem is finding out which of these is the cause. If your baby has not fed for a couple of hours then he is probably due for a feed – problem solved. If he seems unsettled following a feed he may have wind – even breastfed babies do get wind. Winding him can solve this problem. Obviously, if you haven't changed his nappy recently, then try this and it may solve the problem.

Q. My baby seems to want non-stop feeding, especially in the early evening.

Some babies, even after feeding, winding and changing still don't settle easily. Often this happens at a particular time of day. Generally the 'fussy' time tends to be early evening – usually this coincides with you needing to sort out the tea for the rest of the family, or to deal with other children. Perhaps your baby can pick up on the fact that you are more stressed and anxious at this time; consequently he doesn't settle. Another effect of you being more anxious is that it can inhibit your letdown reflex. This will result in your baby getting less milk than he otherwise would.

By the early evening you have probably been busy through the day and not had the opportunity to rest – this can also affect your milk quality, which in turn may mean your baby feels less satisfied following his feed. If this is the case, and it is difficult to change your routine, then you may just need to accept that your new baby is picking up on your signals and try to give him some attention.

It may help if you can carry your baby close to you – remember, skin-to-skin contact is not just for birth, it can be very helpful in calming your baby at these times. If you have a baby carrier, wear it in front of you so he is against your chest and so can hear your heartbeat and feel and smell your closeness.

If this behaviour happens more than just once a day, perhaps at a particular time, then you need to look at how you are responding to your baby. It may be that this is happening after your baby has breastfed himself to sleep and then awakens shortly afterwards, so you offer a further feed. It is quite normal that if your baby is unsettled you will try to feed, wind and change and if he continues not to settle then there is a temptation to repeat this process. However, this can create a cycle that can then be difficult to break. So, if you have fed baby and winded him and checked for/changed a wet/dirty nappy then you should try to get your baby to sleep rather than feeding him again. Many babies feel comforted by being swaddled, so you could try this – just don't wrap him too tightly and don't swaddle him on a hot day.

Tips for getting your baby to sleep

Most parents try to get baby to sleep by either rocking him or putting him over one shoulder and walking round until he falls asleep. This can be very tiring, especially if it happens in the middle of the night. Also, when baby is then laid down on his back he will often wake again soon afterwards.

Sitting down and stroking your baby

Try sitting comfortably, perhaps listening to some music (this can be calming for both you and baby). Lie baby over your lap on his tummy and either pat or stroke his back gently. Continue this until baby is asleep, when you can then try to transfer him back into his cot/basket.

Womb noises

There are some cassette tapes and CD which play noises that represent 'womb noises' – some contain muffled voices and whooshing noises, similar to a washing machine. Some babies respond well to this 'womb music' and settle to sleep while listening to it. This tends to work best if you have introduced the music in the early weeks. It can be used during the day or at night – and actually can be relaxing for parents too, and can help to bring about a feeling of sleepiness for both you and baby.

Turn on the washing machine

During the day you may find the washing machine (when it is running) or a very quiet radio useful. These can help lull your baby off to sleep. Again, this is often more successful in the first two to three months.

Go for a walk

If your baby is older than this and is regularly unsettled, try taking him for a walk in his pushchair (suitably dressed).

Go for a drive

Another option is to go for a drive in the car. This is often so successful that you may find yourself driving no more than a few metres before baby is asleep – a very useful ploy, although it may not seem quite so appealing in the middle of the night!

Try massage

Another helpful solution is to introduce a baby massage into your routine. You can do this whenever it suits you, so it may be following a morning bath or during the evening, incorporating it into the bedtime routine. If your baby tends to be unsettled at a particular time of day then try to use baby massage around that time. Baby massage is less likely to be successful when your baby is very unsettled, crying or hungry.

It is worth trying to start introducing baby massage into your daily routine in the early days, as this becomes an enjoyable time for both you and baby. This will in itself then become a relaxing time and will lead to your baby becoming used to this calm atmosphere. You can read more about baby massage in *Teach Yourself Baby Massage and Yoga* (Hodder Education).

Including baby massage in your routine

- You should lay your baby on the floor, on a towel on the carpet.
- Make sure the room is free of draughts and is warm, especially if your baby is still quite young.
- You do not need to use any special products, as baby oils can often be too greasy. A small amount of oil such as grapeseed oil (which is widely available) will be suitable.
- Have your baby completely undressed, but you may wish to keep the nappy on, just in case!
- Your baby may not be happy about being on his tummy in the early days, so you may wish to start with him on his back, looking at you. Once he is used to the massage, you can start by gently stroking upwards over the back area, with baby lying on his tummy.
- Talk to your baby quietly and soothingly as you do this massage.
- When massaging the tummy area, use very gentle strokes, going round in a clockwise direction over the tummy – this has been shown to help babies with colic.
- Massage the arms and legs by putting your hand gently around the limb and then, with a gentle back and forward motion, massage down the arm or leg.
- If you decide to do this before bath time, make sure you do not use too much oil and be careful how you hold baby when bathing him. Your hands can be quite greasy which can make it difficult to hold on to him securely.

Q. My baby seems to fall asleep after just a few minutes on the breast, then wakes frequently in between.

If your baby is falling asleep while he should still be feeding then this needs to be stopped as it is likely to lead to sore nipples.

Your baby should only be offered the breast if he has woken for a feed, so presumably he is hungry! If he then seems to doze off, sit him up as if you were trying to wind him. The action of sitting him up may rouse him a little. Change the position you are using to feed him – some babies tend to fall asleep more when held in the cradle hold, so try feeding him in a rugby-ball hold instead.

If he starts to drop off, stroke his cheek to stimulate him to suckle again, or give your breast a little jiggle while still in his mouth, just to remind him it is still there! It may be that your baby is using your breast as a 'dummy', merely sucking himself back to sleep; this can lead to sleep problems for your baby and sore nipples for you.

Ensure that your baby is hungry before you start to breastfeed. When he is breastfeeding, if he stops, then use your hand to compress your breast, as if you are expressing your breast milk. This will squeeze some milk into your baby's mouth and encourage him to continue to suckle.

Crying

An unsettled baby may spend quite some time crying, so look over the advice in the previous section.

One of the problems you have, as a new mother, is to work out why your baby is crying – and this may not be as easy as it would seem. Some babies will cry for between one and three hours a day anyway, although not necessarily in one long sequence. If your baby is hungry he will usually cry, but this does not mean that every time he cries he is hungry. Your baby will cry for lots of other reasons – it is the only way he has to communicate with you and let you know he needs something, especially in the early days.

So if he is tired, or over-tired, has wind, a dirty nappy, is too hot or too cold, bored or has has been over-stimulated he will cry. On most occasions if your baby cries and you put him to the breast he will suckle and appear to feed; however, it may be that your baby is using your breast simply as a comforter and so may settle and fall asleep quite quickly as a result of being calmed and soothed. This may mean that he develops the habit of not being able to fall asleep unless he is 'on your breast'.

Why is my baby crying?

- He may be hungry – this will usually be preceded by hunger cues (see Chapter 03).
- He may be in pain.
- He may be bored.
- He may be tired, over-tired or uncomfortable.
- He may be ill – but an ill baby will usually have other symptoms such as a temperature, diarrhoea, being lethargic or not being interested in feeding.

Tips to try if your baby is crying

If your baby is crying and you have fed him recently, winded him and changed his nappy – what do you do now?

Put him down for a nap

I would suggest that you attempt to put him down for a rest, unless the crying is of the screaming variety. Listen to his cry; it may be more of a tired whine, than a scream.

Hold him close

Some babies do like to be held close to you for a while. Remember, your baby has been inside you for nine months during which he could hear your voice and heartbeat – suddenly that comfort has gone. A very young baby will not necessarily know you are close by, although when he is slightly older he may be able to see you are close by and be comforted by that. Don't worry about spoiling him by carrying him around or cuddling/rocking him. Ignoring him and leaving him to cry may simply result in both of you feeling emotionally exhausted very quickly.

Keep calm

Try to keep calm yourself – this is very difficult when your baby is relentless in his crying. If you have had a day packed full of visitors your baby may just be very tired from being over-stimulated. Remove yourself and your baby, go and sit somewhere quiet, or with some music playing quietly in the background. Talk calmly and soothingly to your baby. If he has not been fed for a couple of hours, it may be that he *is* hungry, so try to offer the breast during this time, remembering that if he has been crying for a long period he may be prone to wind and this may mean he brings up some feed if you don't wind him at the end.

Try swaddling

Then put your baby into his cot/crib/Moses basket. He may like being swaddled, so try this – but not too tight. Put him on his back, feet to the bottom of the cot/crib. You may want to try some 'white noise', so turning on the vacuum cleaner or hairdryer can be quite soothing.

Ask for help

If all else fails and you have tried the suggestions above and those for coping with an unsettled baby, then ask for some help from your partner or a good friend. Just have a little time to yourself, away from the crying – where you can relax, listen to some music or just sit quietly, take some deep breaths and calm down. Listening to your baby crying for a long period of time is very draining and, if you cannot seem to soothe your baby, you will inevitably become more anxious and agitated yourself. This will transmit to your baby and may affect your milk letdown by inhibiting oxytocin production.

There is also a national helpline you can ring – CRYSIS – contact details for which can be found in 'Taking it further'. There may be other more local self-help networks – again some details are be listed in 'Taking it further'. Do also speak to your midwife or health visitor.

This advice is given assuming that your baby is otherwise well. If your baby's cry is different, for instance is high-pitched, or if he is lethargic, has a temperature or appears ill (trust your judgement) you should contact your doctor.

If your baby is crying/unsettled:

- Determine if he is hungry, wet/dirty or has wind.
- Hold him close – let him hear your heartbeat. Try a baby carrier/sling or skin-to-skin contact.
- Rock baby to soothe him, perhaps with some quiet music playing.
- Sit with baby lying over your lap, stroking or patting his back.
- Try gentle baby massage.
- Give your baby a warm bath, then swaddle him and wrap him snugly in a soft blanket.
- Stay calm and talk to him in a soothing way.
- Let him listen to a continuous noise, such as the washing machine, vacuum cleaner or womb-music recording.

- Older babies may enjoy lying on a mat – kicking their legs or just watching what you are doing.
- Resort to taking baby for a walk in his pushchair or for a drive in the car.
- Ask for help from a friend/partner to just have some time away and relax yourself.
- Phone a friend, a breastfeeding counsellor, CRYSIS, or other support network; speak to your midwife or health visitor.

Vomiting or reflux?

Q. My baby is being sick and bringing back his feed. What should I do?

Is your baby bringing his feeds back? Is he vomiting or is this just reflux? How do you tell the difference? See below to find out more about vomiting and reflux and the difference between them.

Reflux

Reflux may make your baby vomit, but due to a very specific reason. It can occur in babies from a couple of weeks old and can last some considerable time, even past his first birthday. It happens when the muscle around the neck of the stomach (which keeps it closed) is not fully developed. Normally as milk enters the stomach and mixes with acid to begin digestion, this muscle tightens to prevent any regurgitation of milk back up into the gullet. In some babies, this muscle relaxes instead of tightening which allows the milk and some of the acid content to return and this can irritate the lining of the gullet. Sometimes your baby will seem to bring this back up, or it may just irritate the gullet or back of the throat and not actually be spat up, but may cause some discomfort. So you may notice your baby regurgitates a little milk following his feed or he may develop hiccups after he has fed.

Sometimes reflux happens because the feed has not been managed correctly, so look at the position you hold baby in, especially if giving a bottle, or the amount of feed being taken. If you think your baby is suffering from reflux, try to feed him in as upright a position as possible and keep him in a 'sitting position' for at least half an hour following the feed, to try to help keep the milk in his stomach. When you do put him in his cot/crib, put something under the head of the mattress to prop it up, such as a rolled up towel or blanket.

Reflux usually includes some regurgitation, but in some babies there may be none at all, just a baby who seems distressed on feeding – this is due to milk reflux into the gullet which can cause a burning sensation. This may be enough to put your baby off his feed, so if he is crying and showing signs of distress during the feed, reflux may be the cause. If this problem continues you should discuss it with your doctor. If reflux is the cause he will be able to prescribe something such as Gaviscon, to help prevent it. In most cases this will help resolve the problem.

Try to continue to breastfeed, as your breast milk is easily digested and therefore less irritating to the gullet. Where you can, avoid caffeine in your diet as this seems to be linked with reflux in some cases.

Reflux could be happening as a result of overfeeding – he is taking in too much milk for the size of his small stomach. It may just be because he is greedy, or if you have an abundant milk supply that he simply keeps taking! So if your baby does seem to feed and feed before bringing back (what seems to be) a large part of it, it is quite likely that he is just overfeeding and his stomach rejects the excess.

Vomiting due to overfeeding – Katie's experience

Katie was breastfeeding Jack, her first baby, very successfully. She knew she was producing more than adequate amounts of breast milk as she found her breasts leaking milk during the night and first thing in the morning, despite the fact that she was feeding Jack at least twice during the night. Her breasts were very full prior to feeding and Jack attached to the breast and fed well.

She spoke to me because she was concerned that Jack was 'vomiting' after some feeds. When I asked her to describe this, it was apparent that Jack was being overfed, simply because Katie had such an abundant supply of milk. The vomiting was actually reflux, as Jack rejected the excess milk his stomach simply could not retain. Jack was otherwise well and healthy and gaining weight extremely well, so I was not concerned that this was a sign of something more severe. Also, the 'vomiting' did not happen at every feed but tended to be more likely to follow a breastfeed when Katie had noticed her breast milk flowing very well and Jack was almost gagging on the amount of milk available.

He also had frequent dirty nappies with a frothy greenish stool, which often accompany an over-production of breast milk.

I advised Katie to try to feed Jack only from one breast at each feed in order that he took more high-fat hind milk, which would satisfy him sooner. If he seemed to be gagging on the flow, Katie could also express a little milk first, in order to reduce the amount of fast-flowing fore milk Jack was taking.

As Jack grew, this became less of a problem, and Katie's milk supply adjusted to the Jack's demand, so she did not continue to 'leak' milk.

Vomiting

Vomiting can occur without being related to reflux. This can be anything from a small amount of milk (possetting) to a full explosive amount. During the first few weeks of baby's life a small amount of vomiting is quite normal as he adjusts to his feeding pattern. If he is overfeeding then you may notice that he brings back a sizable volume of his feed, but continues to gain weight. Look for the other signs of such as the type and colour of his stools. So your baby may vomit for reasons other than due to reflux, but this will not be associated with any other signs of distress in your baby; so although he may bring some of the feed back, he is unlikely to be crying or upset by this.

Occasionally your baby may vomit following feeds in the first day or two and this may be related to him having swallowed some of the contents of your amniotic fluid, which may be upsetting him. You may also see streaks of mucous in his vomit – tell your midwife about this as she will be able to advise you on what to do. In most cases this will settle down on its own.

If you breastfeed your baby after he has been crying for a while, he may vomit. This is because there may be a pocket of air trapped in his stomach, so when the wind is brought up it will also bring back part of the feed. This is not really a true vomit. Again, your midwife or health visitor will be able to discuss with you if it is a case of reflux or if your baby really is vomiting regularly. If it is the latter she will be able to tell you if there is any reason for concern.

If your baby does vomit very forcefully, shooting the vomit out of his mouth, you need to speak to your doctor. It may be due to pyloric stenosis, which is when the muscle between the stomach and the gut is thickened and causes a blockage. It tends to appear at around two to three weeks of age and you may notice that your baby also seems constipated. This is more common in boys and is easily treated with surgery.

The best way of dealing with post-feed vomiting and reflux is always to have a towel, bib or cotton nappy close by. When your baby has finished his breastfeed, put this around your lap, or on your shoulder, and wind him. But remember, if your baby is otherwise well, happy and healthy it is unlikely that there is any sinister cause behind the vomiting.

Constipation

Q. How many times a day should my baby be passing a stool?

Your breastfed baby may not have many dirty nappies and, when well-established on the breast, some babies may only pass a stool once or twice a week. Other breastfed infants may dirty their nappy several times a day – it depends very much on the individual, particularly in the first few weeks. There is little waste from your breast milk as it is so easily and well-absorbed by your baby. So it can be quite normal for your baby not to have a dirty nappy more than every few days, providing this is a soft stool and he seems happy.

If your baby passes a stool that is hard and looks more like small pellets then this is seen as constipation. It is very uncommon for a breastfed baby to experience this problem. It is far more common in bottle-fed babies, although it is still unlikely in the first three months. It is more likely once your baby has started to take solids, in which case you may need to increase his fluid intake, offering him some water in between feeds.

Your baby's first stool is thick and tar-like; if your baby does not pass this stool you will need to tell your midwife. Following this the stool should start to change as he takes in milk; if this does not seem to be happening, again you should tell your midwife or doctor, as this could indicate a problem or suggest that your baby is not getting enough milk. Most babies who are exclusively breastfed will have quite frequent stools up to about six weeks of age, when they may become less frequent but should remain soft. If this is the case and your baby is gaining weight there is little to worry about.

Your baby may appear to be grunting or straining prior to his dirty nappy, but this does not necessarily mean he is constipated. In the past, suggestions to overcome constipation included adding brown sugar to some water, or giving baby some diluted orange or prune juice. These are not recommended as they are not considered suitable for young babies (less than six months old).

What your baby's stool should look like

- His first stool (meconium) will be thick and tar-like. It will appear black or very dark green.
- His changing stool should be greenish-yellow and grainy. You will see this around day 3 or 4. It is a good sign that your baby is getting your breast milk.
- Normal breastfed stool is usually yellow or mustard coloured, possibly grainy.
- Normal breastfed stools do not smell nasty; in fact there is often a particular sweetish smell to them.
- Diarrhoea is frequent, watery and greener than usual.
- Constipated stool is hard and pellet-like.
- Overfeeding stools are frequent and frothy green.

Colic

Q. What is colic?

The definition of colic is 'crying lasting more than three hours a day, for more than three days a week, lasting more than three weeks'. It is a term often given to a baby who seems to be crying incessantly, particularly in the early evening, and cannot be soothed and calmed. Science is yet to agree on an explanation for colic. There is a view that it may be associated with trapped wind, but this has not been proven.

Colic tends to affect babies under three months of age, and is often worst at around six to eight weeks of age. In most cases, the baby seems to grow out of it after they reach three months old. However, in the meantime this is a very testing time for you, as the parents.

You may notice your baby pulling up his legs towards his stomach during this time, and the crying is more of the screaming variety which makes it sound as if your baby is in great distress. You may notice that your baby seems in pain after feeds or before he dirties his nappy.

Some things to bear in mind when trying to decide if your baby has colic:

- Think whether your baby had been crying for a long time before his feed. If he has, he may have swallowed a lot of air and this can cause him discomfort.
- If he has taken a bottle recently, was he gulping and taking air in at the same time?
- Look over the advice given earlier in the chapter on unsettled and crying babies, and try the suggestions given there for soothing or distracting your baby.
- Colic is usually self-limiting and it will pass, although this is of little comfort to you when trying to cope with it daily. Try to stay calm, although this is not easy when your baby won't stop screaming. However, just remember that it will pass!

Q. Could my baby be allergic to my something in my breast milk?

If your baby seems particularly troubled after a feed, think about what you have eaten in the hours prior to the last feed. If you are bottle-feeding your baby you may be tempted to change the milk product you are giving but, in most cases, this will have little effect.

Few babies are actually allergic to or intolerant of any of the food you are eating, although there will be a small number for whom this is a problem. If you notice an increase in colic symptoms in your breastfed baby following a feed, can you relate this to something you have eaten? It may be that you have eaten foods that are linked with creating 'windiness', such as cauliflower, cabbage or some spices. If you have eaten any of these foods they may have passed through your milk to your baby, which can lead to wind and this may give your baby colic symptoms. Avoid these foods for a while and see if things improve. Try them again at a later date and see how your baby reacts. A very small number of babies are allergic to or intolerant of dairy products and may display colic symptoms after feeding when you have eaten some of these. You will find advice regarding this in the next section, on milk intolerance/allergy.

If you have tried the suggestions for settling your baby there are some products available to relieve colic that you may wish to try.

Your doctor could prescribe an antispasmodic mixture, which is designed to ease the pain and discomfort of colic. There are some homeopathic remedies also available, such as Camomilla, which you will find at your local health food shop or some chemists. This is available in liquid drop form or in granules (which may also be recommended for teething).

Dealing with your baby with colic

- Try carrying your baby around with you, skin-to-skin or in a baby carrier, across your chest.
- Put your baby over your lap, or carry him round lying 'tummy down' over your arms.
- Try swaddling or wrapping your baby snugly.
- Rule out any obvious reasons for his distress, such as hunger or a dirty nappy.
- Look to see if there is a pattern in any foods you have eaten or given to baby. Write down what you have eaten. Does the colic seem worse at certain times of day or after some feeds? What have you eaten in the previous four to six hours?
- Homeopathic remedies are available for colic.
- Your doctor may prescribe a preparation such as Gaviscon or Infacol.

Milk intolerance/allergy

Some people believe that milk intolerance or allergy has become a fashionable diagnosis, one with little basis. It is certainly true that incidence varies widely depending on whether it is based on self-reporting or as a result of an objective 'food challenge'. A number of adults (around one in five) believe themselves to have a food allergy, but actual testing puts that figure much lower, at 1 per cent of adults and 1 to 2 per cent of children. Food intolerance is thought to affect between 5 and 8 per cent of children and 1 to 2 per cent of adults.

Food intolerance is a general term to describe an unwanted reaction to a particular foodstuff or ingredient, in this case milk. An allergy is a particular type of intolerance which actually involves a response within the immune system, so that a specific food substance is seen as 'foreign' and causes the release of antibodies in the body. This triggers a response from other cells in the body, leading to inflammation and a range of other symptoms. This type of reaction tends to happen immediately and on each occasion that the offending foodstuff is eaten.

Some food allergies, including that to milk, may be outgrown, usually by the age of three years old. Other allergies, such as to peanuts, are usually life long. Symptoms can be extreme, as in anaphylaxis, but more commonly babies and children with (milk) intolerance can display a range of symptoms, including gastro-intestinal upsets (vomiting, colic, diarrhoea), respiratory problems such as asthma, a runny nose (rhinitis) or catarrh, skin reactions (urticaria or eczema) or even some behavioural problems such as hyperactivity.

Lactose intolerance

Lactose (milk sugar) needs to be broken down in a baby's body by a particular enzyme (lactase). If there is not enough of this enzyme in the body then this cannot happen, so the milk sugar will not be absorbed. This means it will pass straight through the gut into the large intestine and so lead to bloating, flatulence, diarrhoea and abdominal pain and discomfort.

Lactose intolerance is more common in certain groups of people, particularly those from South-East Asia, the Middle East, India and some parts of Africa. Although it can occur in anyone as a temporary condition, this is usually due to a gastric upset, which may prevent the bowel being able to absorb correctly for a period of time.

Milk protein allergy

This is much less common than lactose intolerance but is more likely to be found in children than adults, although most will grow out of it in time. All cows' milk protein has to be excluded from their diet. Obviously if your baby is on formula milk then a substitute has to be found and you will need to discuss this with your doctor and midwife/health visitor. It is not something you should just decide without medical supervision, partly because babies who are allergic to cows' milk protein may also be allergic to the protein found in some other substitutes, such as soya milk and goat's milk.

However, this can also be a problem if your baby is being breastfed, when milk protein from your diet is passed through to your baby in your breast milk. If this is the case then you need to have a dairy-free diet while you are breastfeeding. Initially this can be quite difficult to follow and still maintain a healthy balanced diet, as milk protein is found in many other foods, not just milk or obvious dairy products.

Q. My baby seems to be crying all the time. Could he be allergic to my breast milk?

In some cases babies may be more prone to colic when there is a higher amount of cows' milk protein in the breast milk, so it may be worth trying to exclude this as a cause of colic if your baby does seem to be affected. You need to exclude all cows' milk protein from your diet for a week and see if there is any improvement in your baby's symptoms. If there is a difference then you should speak to your doctor who can then confirm the diagnosis and give you some expert advice on your own diet in order that this is not too restrictive. It can be quite difficult to follow such a restrictive diet as milk protein is often a 'hidden' substance in many foods (even some crisps, baked beans etc.), so you will need to look closely at the label of everything you buy. However, if your baby does show signs of cows' milk allergy while you are breastfeeding it may be necessary to exclude this from your diet throughout the time you are breastfeeding.

Signs to look for if you think your baby is allergic to milk protein:

- colic-like symptoms
- excessive crying, especially if this happens during or shortly after breastfeeding
- loose stools; may have mucous in them
- rashes or eczema
- wheeziness
- snuffly nose
- vomiting.

It will be important to keep this intolerance in mind when you commence weaning as it is necessary to ensure that your baby still receives a balanced diet. An attempt to reintroduce small amounts of cows' milk protein back into the diet can be planned so that any effects can be monitored. This may not be until he is older, perhaps after his first birthday.

Jaundice

Jaundice is when the baby's skin looks yellow and the whites of his eyes may also look slightly yellow. It is quite common and most babies will have a small amount of jaundice, which starts after the first 24 hours, reaches a peak around day 3 or 4 and then gradually fades over the next week to ten days. Some breastfed babies do have slightly higher levels of jaundice.

This jaundice (known as physiological jaundice) occurs as a result of the breakdown products from blood (bilirubin) not being excreted, and is quite normal in most newborn babies. It is usually self-limiting and tends to happen while your baby's body is still trying to cope with breaking down and getting rid of these products. Obviously while you were pregnant you did all this for your baby, as your baby's waste would have been passed to you via the umbilical cord. When your baby is born he suddenly has to take over all of these functions and it can take a few days for his body to adjust and be able to deal with everything.

Also, while you were pregnant your baby had a lot of red blood cells (which help pass all your nutrients to him), so all of these have to be broken down and excreted once he is born. If your baby is born prematurely then he may take even longer to adjust to this while his body completes its development and carries out these important functions, so jaundice may last longer. Usually no treatment is necessary.

If your baby is bruised following delivery, perhaps following a forceps delivery, this can mean that he may be more affected by jaundice as his body has to deal with the extra blood cells.

The pigment, bilirubin, will also be in your baby's first stool, the meconium. The sooner this is excreted by your baby the better, as the bilirubin can be reabsorbed and re-circulated, which can lead to an increase in jaundice.

Q. My baby is jaundiced. What can I do?

You can help to prevent or reduce the impact and level of jaundice by frequently breastfeeding, although this can sometimes be difficult as a jaundiced baby is often quite sleepy and so difficult to feed.

It is important to feed your baby as soon after delivery as possible and then as often as he wants, for as long as he wants. Remember, colostrum acts as a laxative and so will help stimulate your baby to excrete the meconium, reducing the amount of bilirubin available for reabsorption.

Feed as frequently as possible, as both colostrum and breast milk contain fat that helps to stimulate your baby's bowel. Do not be tempted to give your baby extra drinks, especially of water. In the past this was thought to be helpful in 'washing' the jaundice out of the system, but very little bilirubin is excreted in the urine. A large proportion is excreted in the stool so it is more important that your baby takes extra breast milk.

If your baby is sleepy and not feeding very well, express your breast milk in between feeds and try to give this to baby following his next breastfeed to ensure he takes as much milk as possible.

Physiological jaundice

- This is a very common condition that tends to happen around 24–48 hours after delivery, peaks around 4 or 5 days and resolves spontaneously.
- Try to feed frequently and as early as possible after delivery to encourage passage of the first stool.
- Colostrum has a laxative effect and assists baby to pass his first stool (meconium).
- Jaundiced babies tend to be sleepy, which can be exaggerated if you had pain relief in labour, especially pethidine.
- It may be necessary to encourage your baby to feed frequently rather than waiting for him to 'demand feed'.
- Phototherapy may be necessary in some cases. If so, baby should receive frequent feeds in order to prevent any dehydration.
- If your baby is not waking regularly for feeds, try giving him extra expressed breast milk following his feed or use a lactation aid to increase the amount he takes during his feed.

Breast milk jaundice

Late-onset jaundice, which seems to happen suddenly towards the end of the first week, when your baby has been getting your breast milk, can be known as 'breast milk jaundice'. Jaundice in these babies seems to last longer – sometimes up to a month or six weeks old. Although this can be worrying for you, it is not very serious and actually isn't dangerous for your baby and, although it tends to last longer, the levels of jaundice don't get too high.

It is often difficult to prove that the jaundice is related to breastfeeding, and usually this is only identified when all other tests prove there is no other cause, and if jaundice is due to other causes there will be other signs. The only real way of finding out is to stop breastfeeding for a couple of days and see whether the jaundice levels drop. However, don't be tempted to give up breastfeeding just to 'prove' this is the problem. It doesn't help breastfeeding itself, and in some cases giving your baby glucose water instead of breastfeeding actually seems to make it worse, not better. If nothing else can be found to be the problem, don't worry too much about it. You will find your baby is otherwise alert and feeding well and as he grows you will find it will start to clear up as he is able to deal with it better.

Very occasionally, if the levels of jaundice do become very high, your doctor may ask you to stop breastfeeding for a while and give your baby a supplement, probably of formula milk. At this point the jaundice levels often tend to fall, and when you do recommence breastfeeding, they don't seem to reach the same high levels again. If it is suggested to you that you stop breastfeeding for a while, it is better if you can express your breast milk when your baby would have gone to the breast so that you maintain your supply. If this is only for a couple of feeds then there shouldn't be too much effect on your milk supply.

A diagnosis of breast milk jaundice should not be made until other, more serious forms of jaundice are ruled out. But it is possible to exclude other causes without needing to interrupt breastfeeding. In the past it was more common to advise suspending breastfeeding as it could quickly confirm the diagnosis; however, it is not usually necessary and doesn't help successful breastfeeding in the long term.

Phototherapy

Q. My jaundiced baby has been put under some ultra-violet lights. What does this do and can I do anything to help reduce the jaundice?

If your baby does develop jaundice while you are in hospital it may be suggested that he is 'put under the lights' (this is also known as phototherapy treatment). Sunlight helps to break down the bilirubin pigment so can help to reduce the level of jaundice in your baby. Ultraviolet lights act in the same way, so putting baby near the window if it is a sunny day will also help.

If your baby has physiological jaundice it will resolve on its own, but is often helped by the use of phototherapy. If your baby does have phototherapy he will need to be undressed, except for his nappy, with his eyes covered (as the light can damage the eyes). Sometimes this can mean babies lose more fluid than usual, which can add to their sleepiness and may lead to diarrhoea, which can result in a sore bottom. So the more you can feed your baby the better, and collecting expressed milk to give to him will also help.

Try to breastfeed as often as you can, although you may find your baby is sleepier. If this is the case, you can express your breast milk in between feeds; this will help increase your milk supply and you can then give this milk to your baby if necessary.

The Sleepy Baby

Q. My baby is quite sleepy after delivery and not really interested in breastfeeding. What can I do?

Your baby may be sleepy because you had some pain relief while you were in labour. This may mean he is less interested in feeding immediately after delivery and it can also affect the first few days of breastfeeding; this is especially true if you received pethidine shortly before delivery. This drug will make you sleepy and will pass through to your baby during labour; then when you start breastfeeding your baby will receive some more of the drug via your breast milk.

If your baby is quite sleepy due to pethidine being administered during delivery then you may need to be more vigilant in ensuring your baby feeds as often as possible because, to some extent, he is 'sedated' and therefore will not display normal behaviour, such as waking for feeds regularly.

If you have skin-to-skin contact straight after delivery, this may help your baby to show more interest in feeding. Let your baby lie undisturbed on your tummy until he is seems ready to make the attempt to latch himself on to the breast. If left there for long enough, your baby will attempt to reach your breast and try to latch himself on. Sometimes this is less successful when the process is stopped, perhaps because he is only left on your tummy for too short a time (less than 20 minutes) before being taken to be weighed and measured. If you can leave your baby on your tummy until he has had the opportunity to try and latch himself on to the breast this could help to stimulate him.

You could use a lactation aid (see Chapter 05) which can help to increase the amount of milk your baby can take during the feed. If you can express some breast milk, then your baby can breastfeed while also receiving the extra expressed milk at the same time. This can help to ensure he is getting enough milk and nutrients. It also builds up and maintains your supply.

There are a number of other problems that may lead to difficulties and prevent your baby from breastfeeding successfully. Fortunately these are quite rare, but need to be kept in mind in order to overcome the problems. One particular problem that can affect breastfeeding and lead to speech difficulties is 'tongue-tie'.

Tongue-tie (ankyloglossia)

This is when the membrane (frenulum) which holds the tongue to the base of the mouth is so tight that it restricts the movement of the tongue. It can prevent the baby from extending his tongue over the lower gum, which can then affect how well he can attach to the breast. The membrane may be a thin attachment or quite thick, becoming thicker as baby gets older.

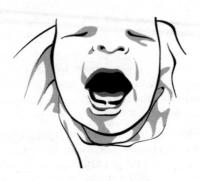

figure 7.1 a baby with tongue-tie

Q. How can tongue-tie affect my feeding?

If the membrane is so tight that baby cannot extend his tongue over the lower gum or form a 'scoop' shape around the areola of the breast, he may have problems attaching and staying on during a breastfeed. While breastfeeding, baby's tongue has to 'milk' the breast tissue; if it is too restricted, this may not be possible for your baby to do. Your baby is also likely to have problems is staying on the breast. If this is not dealt with then your baby will be dissatisfied, not get enough milk and not gain weight.

Tongue-tie – Sara's story

Sara had her second baby, Jack, having breastfed her first baby quite successfully. During the first couple of days, whenever Jack attempted to latch on to the breast, he seemed to go on initially, but then after one or two sucks would slide off. Sara was also beginning to get sore nipples as a result of Jack not being attached properly.

When I looked in Jack's mouth it was possible to see that the membrane was attached almost at the tip of the tongue, which meant he could not stick his tongue out to form a scoop to take in the areola tissue of the breast. Once this membrane was cut, he was put straight on to the breast to feed and immediately Sara noticed a difference. He stayed on the breast and fed well, coming off on his own, sleepy and satisfied.

Q. Does tongue-tie cause any other problems?

If left alone, the membrane will usually stretch to allow the tongue to move normally. However sometimes, if this is insufficient, it may affect speech development.

It can also be a problem for babies who bottle-feed as they cannot make a good seal around the teat, so they tend to dribble a lot of the feed out of the side of their mouth and, because this 'seal' is leaky, baby can be very windy as he takes in more air during the feed. The feed can also be prolonged as baby cannot suck efficiently.

If the membrane does not stretch or is not separated, there may be problems when introducing lumpy food, as the tongue will not be able to move the food to the back of the mouth.

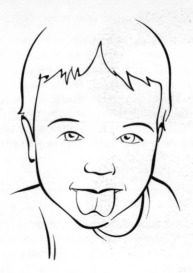

figure 7.2 an older child with unresolved tongue-tie

Q. Can anything be done to help with toungue-tie?

It is becoming more common for the tongue-tie to be separated, sooner rather than later. It is best done in the younger baby, preferably before eight months and, if it is causing problems with breastfeeding, is often carried out within the first couple of weeks. It does not seem to be very painful and in fact a number of babies sleep through the whole procedure. If the procedure is not performed until the child is older, then a local anaesthetic would be used. It must be undertaken by a trained health professional.

When tongue-tie is resolved by cutting the membrane, baby is wrapped up and his head held steady while a trained midwife or doctor uses a sharp pair of blunt-ended scissors to divide the membrane (frenulum). There may be a small amount of bleeding but often there is none and your baby will be put on your breast immediately after the procedure. Often you will feel the difference straight away, in that your baby achieves a much better position and you feel less pain, if any. There are few – if any – side effects for your baby, although occasionally a small white patch may be seen under the tongue for 24–48 hours afterwards and occasionally some babies have a small ulcer, but this is unusual.

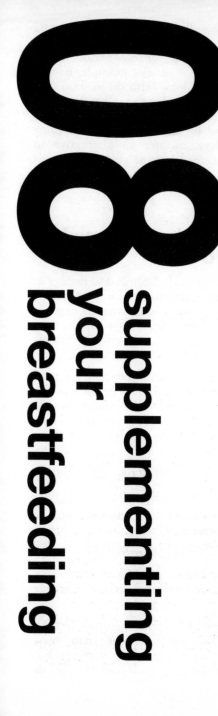

08

supplementing your breastfeeding

In this chapter you will learn:
• about alternative types of milk
• the differences between the types of milk
• whether these are suitable for your baby
• how to make up a formula feed safely
• about sterilization.

Breast milk is the most suitable milk for your baby; Chapter 02 outlines the advantages that breast milk has over formula (cows') milk. However, you may decide, for some reason, to give your baby an alternative form of milk. For example, if your baby is born early or is ill following his birth the medical staff of the neonatal unit may recommend using other forms of feeding initially. Also, if your baby is too preterm or ill he may not be able to breastfeed, and he may need to be fed using different methods. If you have to use an alternative to breastfeeding you may be concerned because your baby shows signs of allergy to or intolerance of cows' milk. This chapter will look at what else you could safely give your baby.

How your baby's development might affect how he is fed

The way your baby needs feeding might be linked to the age at which he is born, as well as his ability to feed. If your baby is born prematurely he may not be able to suck strongly enough, initially, to meet his nutritional needs. So, if your baby is born very early, he may need to receive all his food directly into his bloodstream by intravenous fluids.

Usually a baby born under 30 to 32 weeks' gestation will need to be fed using a tube, which may be put into his stomach, either via his nose or directly through his mouth. If he is born between 30 and 32 weeks' gestation he may be able to 'lap' and so may be able to take some milk from a cup (although this may be in addition to nasogastric/tube feeding).

A baby born at about 32 weeks will start to root for the nipple and will be able to to suckle at the breast, although he may tire quickly. From about 34 to 36 weeks a preterm baby can usually take the entire feed from the breast. However, there may still be a need for some supplements at times.

Q. Should I need to supplement my breastfeeding?

The ideal response to this would be 'no'. However, in reality there will be times when giving your baby a supplement may feel like the only answer.

If your baby is born at full term and is otherwise quite healthy then there is no need to give him any fluids other than breast milk, although sometimes you may wonder if it is necessary. For example, if the weather is hot you may think your baby needs extra water. If your baby is jaundiced, it may be suggested that you give him extra fluids (such as water) to help relieve this. If your baby is crying and your milk has not yet 'come in', you may be offered a bottle of formula. However, none of these are really valid reasons. Your baby does not *need* any additional fluids, of any kind, before your milk comes in. In fact, giving him other fluids will often disrupt your breastfeeding; it fills your baby's stomach so he will not require regular breastfeeding. This will mean that the hormone prolactin is not stimulated frequently enough, which can reduce your milk supply. If your baby does not seem to be satisfied following a feed, or is not feeding well, look at the advice in Chapters 04 and 05. If you are worried about your letdown, about whether you have enough milk or about jaundice then look back over the advice given in Chapters 05 and 07.

If you do need to give your baby any other fluids, such as expressed breast milk, you can use other feeding methods such as a cup, bottle, nasogastric tube or supplemental feeding system. Cup feeding is the best method to use when giving a supplement; it is recommended by the Baby Friendly Initiative and is identified within the Ten Steps (see Chapter 11). If your baby does need a 'top-up' after a feed, you could give him expressed breast milk.

However, there may be some instances where you want to give your baby an additional formula feed – perhaps you have twins or really feel you cannot feed your baby sufficiently. In this case, your first step should be to ask for help, from your midwife or perhaps a local breastfeeding support group (such as National Childbirth Trust, La Leche League or the Association of Breastfeeding Mothers) as they may be able to help support you in breastfeeding. Remember why you wanted to breastfeed and perhaps remind yourself of the benefits linked to breastfeeding for both you and your baby.

Other milks

Cows' milk (formula)

Formula milk is now readily available in various forms, ready-to-pour cartons, smaller, individual ready-to-use packs as well as in the traditional powder form. Making a decision as to which milk to use can be difficult – there is such a range to choose from. If you do decide to use a formula milk, speak to your midwife or health visitor as they may be able to help you. However, most formula milks are really basically the same – they all have to comply with government standards and try to match breast milk as closely as possible.

Cows' milk allergy or intolerance seems to be becoming more common, with an increasing number of bottlefed babies seemingly showing some symptoms of this allergy or intolerance. If there is a history within your family of allergies, or other conditions such as eczema or hay fever, your baby may also have a tendency towards developing allergies, although this is not certain.

Giving an occasional supplement of formula (cows') milk to a breastfed infant could risk sensitizing him. If you do decide to give your baby a bottle of formula milk, ensure you make it up correctly – do not be tempted to add extra powder in order to feed your 'hungrier' baby. There are specific formulas that advertise themselves as being suitable for the hungry baby, but these are not really suitable for younger babies. These formulas have a higher casein content which will fill the baby's stomach and are more difficult to digest, so the stomach empties more slowly, resulting in baby feeling fuller for longer.

Q. My baby seems really hungry and my relatives suggest adding rusk or some baby rice to the bottle formula.

It is important that you do not add anything other than milk, such as baby rusk or cereal, to your baby's bottle. Sometimes there is a temptation to thicken the feed in order that your baby lasts longer between feeds, but this can make the consistency too thick for your baby to take easily. Solids (including baby rice and rusk) are not recommended (even added to a bottle) if your baby is less than six months of age.

If you feel that your baby still seems hungry, discuss this with your health visitor – you may need to increase the amount of milk you give him or the frequency of his feeds, or perhaps look at those formulas aimed at the older baby.

If you are breastfeeding then more frequent feeding is the order of the day – the more often you breastfeed the more milk you will produce to meet his demand.

Q. Can I give my baby another form of milk instead of formula cows' milk?

There are alternatives to cows' milk, such as goats' milk or soya milk, but you should think this through carefully and discuss with your doctor the implications of using a formula made from anything other than modified cows' milk.

Goat's milk

Goats' milk is not recommended for young babies, although sometimes it is thought to be useful for babies who are particularly prone to allergies. However, there are some differences in the composition of goats' and cows' milk: goats' milk has more fat, although this is easier to digest; it forms softer curds, more like your breast milk, as the protein part of the milk has less casein. But goats' milk and cows' milk are very similar in their protein composition, so if your baby seems to react to cows' milk protein then it is quite likely he will react to goats' milk as well.

The mineral content of both goats' milk and cows' milk is also similar, but there are some significant differences: goats' milk does have more calcium, potassium, copper, vitamins B6 and A, while cows milk has more vitamin B12 and folic acid. To make goats' milk more suitable for infants and toddlers, it would need to have folic acid added to it, and multivitamins would still need to be given.

If you believe your baby is allergic to cows' milk then it is best to discuss the options with your doctor and a dietician, rather than just switching him onto a goats' milk formula, especially if your child is under one year old.

Soya milk

You may consider giving soya milk formula to your baby if he seems to be allergic to cows' milk. However, again it is not really recommended for babies under the age of six months and should only be given to those under one year on the advice of your doctor. Ordinary soya milks are not suitable for babies as they do not contain the correct nutrients to allow your baby to develop correctly.

Soya formula often contains glucose, which is likely to be responsible for tooth decay. If your baby is thought to be allergic to cows' milk protein it may be suggested that you try this formula. However, this should be on medical advice only and in that case it will be available on prescription. There are also some signs that babies who are allergic to cows' milk may also be allergic to soya, so it may not be the answer to this problem.

Making up a formula feed

Making up a feed must be done accurately, all equipment must be sterilized prior to use and you should wash your hands before starting to prepare a bottle-feed. The proportions to be used will be clearly stated on the packaging, although this is usually one (flat) scoop of powder to 1 ounce (30 ml) of water. The water must be put into the bottle first and then the powder added, otherwise there may be a lower water to powder ratio, which will result in an over-concentrated formula which can be dangerous as your baby can become dehydrated.

- Fill the kettle with fresh water from the tap – do not use bottled water and do not re-boil any water that is already in the kettle as this can concentrate any nitrates that may be in the water.
- The water should be freshly boiled and then left to cool slightly, for no more than 30 minutes – the water should be between 70°C and 90°C. It takes about 25 minutes for a litre of water to cool to this temperature, or 15 minutes for 500 ml. If you use boiling water there is a risk of scalding yourself, and some formulas have a tendency to go lumpy if mixed with very hot water.
- Pour the water into the bottle, to the required level; to make sure this is accurate, stand the bottle on a surface and look at it from the side.
- Then add the correct number of scoops of powder. Always use the scoop provided with that particular formula.
- Do not heap powder on the scoop – level it off, and don't add an extra scoop for luck.
- Then put the lid on the bottle and shake it to help dissolve the powder.
- The feed should then be cooled quickly, by running it under cool water before giving to your baby. It is important to cool the feed quickly as any bacteria in the feed will tend to

multiply rapidly – this happens most rapidly between 7°C and 65°C.

- Any of the feed that is not used within two hours should be thrown away,

Each bottle should be made freshly for each feed; it is no longer recommended that a whole day's feeds are made up in one go and then stored in the fridge. This is because the powdered milk is not sterile when it is made and there is a small risk that it could be contaminated, so if it is then stored as warm milk this provides the perfect conditions for organisms to grow in. It is the length of time for which the prepared feed is stored that increases the risk of micro-organsims multiplying.

Where it is simply not practical to make the feed up freshly, for example if you are going out for a length of time, then there are alternatives. It may be possible to use ready-to-use liquid formula milk, although this can be more expensive if used regularly, for example if you need to provide the feeds for your childminder.

Alternatively, you can carry the boiled water in a sealed vacuum flask (which should be able to keep it at the right temperature) in order to prepare the feed when required. Then you just add this to the bottle before any powder, as you would normally. You may wish to anticipate your baby's night feed by putting some boiled water in a thermos and then mixing it with the powder when he starts to stir for his feed.

Do not store the boiled water in the bottles in the fridge because it will not be hot enough to kill any bacteria in the powder – it must be at least 70°C as, at this temperature, any bacteria are killed almost instantly.

Preparing a formula feed

- Boil fresh water in a kettle and allow it to cool for no more than 30 minutes.
- Use water that is between 70°C and 90°C.
- Use the manufacturer's instructions with regard to the proportion of water to milk powder.
- Put the required amount of water into the bottle before adding the milk powder.
- Always use the scoop provided with the formula milk – do not heap the scoop.

- Shake the mixture to dissolve the powder.
- Cool the bottle quickly under cold running water.
- Any feed not taken within two hours should be discarded.
- Milk should not be made up in advance, but hot boiled water can be stored in a sealed vacuum flask for use later, when the milk powder can be added.

Sterilizing your equipment

All equipment used to prepare your baby's food or bottle, whether this is formula milk, expressed breast milk or introductory solids, must be washed thoroughly and sterilized for all babies under the age of one year.

Wash all the equipment in hot soapy water, using a bottle brush to remove all traces of milk. If you can, turn teats inside out and make sure the hole is completely clear of any milk remnants. Many bottle brushes have a smaller brush at one end which can be used to clean inside the teat.

It is possible to use a chemical sterilizing unit, a steam sterilizer or a microwave steam sterilizer. If you are breastfeeding and just expressing occasionally, you may not wish to purchase any of this specialized equipment with its added expense.

Cold sterilization

Once washed, the cleansed items should then be placed in the sterilizing fluid. It is possible to use chemical sterilization without the need to purchase a particular 'unit'. You can use any tub that has a lid – a bucket or large ice-cream container would be suitable. Just ensure it is deep enough to fully immerse the bottles and equipment.

Keep the container out of the sunlight, or cover it with a cloth, as sunlight can prevent the solution from working effectively. Do not put any metal utensils in the chemical solution as these can become tarnished. When putting any equipment into the container, especially bottles, make sure they do not contain any air bubbles as this area will not be sterilized. Keep all bottles, teats, spoons etc. beneath the level of the fluid to ensure they are properly sterilized. All equipment should be left in the solution undisturbed for at least 30 minutes and the solution should be changed every 24 hours.

Steam/microwave sterilization

Steam sterilization takes about 12 minutes or, if you use a microwave steam sterilizer, about 8 minutes, plus the cooling times. Steam sterilizers kill bateria using steam heat, without the use of any chemicals, and there is no need to rinse bottles after use.

Microwave sterilizers work in a similar way to steam sterilizers, but obviously need to be put in a microwave. This will take around 10 minutes and items will remain sterile for about 3 hours if left in the unit. Remember not to put metal utensils, such as spoons or knives, in a microwave sterilizer. Bear in mind that if you are planning to travel or to visit friends or family, it is worth checking that a microwave will be available. Really, if you are breastfeeding it is not necessary to run to the expense of purchasing such equipment. However, do remember that you will still need to sterilize feeding equipment when you start to introduce mixed feeding on weaning.

Using a supplementer

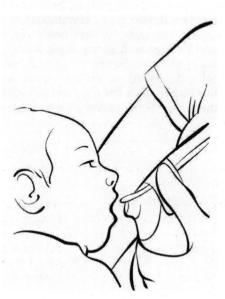

figure 8.1 breastfeeding using a supplementer

A supplemental nursing system (sometimes called a 'Lactaid') can be used to give either your expressed breast milk or formula milk to your baby while he is breastfeeding. This can be used to help induce your lactation if you have not breastfed your baby from birth and then change your mind, or if you have discontinued breastfeeding and wish to re-induce lactation. Some adoptive mothers use this system very successfully.

The amount of milk needed by the baby is put into the bottle, which is worn around the mother's neck. Two very fine feeding tubes that lead from the bottle are laid alongside the nipple and secured to the breast with tape. Then, as the baby suckles at the breast, he will receive the milk from the supplementer, but at the same time he will stimulate the mother's prolactin hormone release and so will assist in the production of breast milk.

The length of time you will need to add milk to the supplementer will obviously depend your baby's age, although as you produce breast milk it may be possible to decrease this amount.

If you are an adoptive mother it is probably fair to say that in most cases you will need to continue to use the supplementer even when you do produce breast milk as, by then, your baby will be older and will need more milk. The amount of milk you produce may not be sufficient for his needs on its own, especially as he will have growth spurts along the way. It can take several weeks to produce the volume of milk required to fully feed your baby, depending on the individual. Sometimes milk will be produced after just a few days and sometimes it can take longer, but the satisfaction you will gain is enormous.

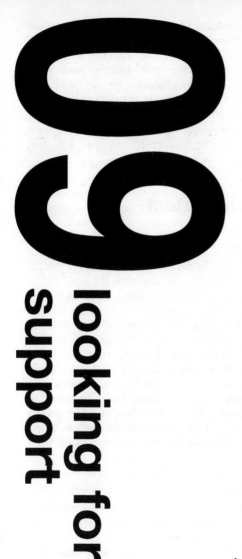

09

looking for support

In this chapter you will learn:
- how support can affect your success in breastfeeding
- the importance of getting emotional support
- the benefit of practical help
- who could be part of your support network.

This chapter is very much focused on identifying the sort of support you may find useful while breastfeeding, so it is perhaps particularly important that you share this chapter with your partner and main supporters, who may include your own mother or your partner's mother. Once they have read this chapter they may feel that they need to read other parts of the book too. If they feel more knowledgeable and confident then, when you feel things are not going so well and you need more support, you will have someone to turn to and they will feel better equipped to give you that support.

Why support is important

Q. Why is support important?

Support from family and friends can influence both the decision to breastfeed and the total duration of the lactation period. Remember that this is *your* decision for *your* baby; family and friends may have different opinions and these can influence how you feel. It is to be hoped that they will be fully supportive of you and your decisions, but keep in mind that, however well-intentioned they are (and it is likely that they will have your best interests at heart), they may have been influenced by other factors which may not necessarily apply to you. For example if, for some reason, a friend was unsuccessful in breastfeeding she may have resorted to bottle-feeding, so she may not be able to fully support you or understand what you are going through when any problems occur. When you are looking for an answer, other than resorting to bottle-feeding, she may not be able to give you any practical tips and may feel ambiguous about breastfeeding in general after her negative experience of it.

Similarly, when your baby is crying in the middle of the night and you are struggling with tiredness, your partner may question whether breastfeeding for every feed is really necessary. He may also be influenced by his own mother, who may have received very different support and information when he was a baby from that given now. Our understanding of how successful breastfeeding occurs has changed and this has affected midwives' practice. So, although in the past new mothers may have been advised to give baby a bottle, it is now recognized that this should be avoided wherever possible as it undermines breastfeeding as well as inducing irreversible changes within the baby's system.

What support might you need?

There are essentially two types of support you are likely to feel you need: practical help and emotional support, both of which are very important in their own way.

How your partner feels about you breastfeeding and how much he supports your decision can influence several aspects of breastfeeding, including the initial decision whether or not to breastfeed, how you undertake and cope with the first feed, how long you breastfeed for and understanding the risks of giving your baby a bottle-feed. If your partner is your main supporter and is involved with your decision, then he can help you when you are feeling a little low and under pressure, particularly in providing emotional support. Sometimes when you are feeling tired or things are not going quite as you expected, you will need this backup. Someone telling you that what you are doing is great and that you are coping wonderfully (whether you feel you are or not) can encourage you and give you back your confidence.

Your relatives may be able to help in this way too. Perhaps your mother or a sister, especially if they breastfed too, could help build up your confidence and inspire you to continue feeding.

How dads can help

As a new mother you are likely to feel exhausted a lot of the time, regardless of whether or not you are breastfeeding. However, many dads will still be going out to work and may be just as exhausted as you as a result of disturbed nights. This disturbed sleep pattern is likely to occur whether or not you are breastfeeding, but is often used to justify stopping breastfeeding, perhaps because it is thought that if you are not breastfeeding your partner could give baby a bottle-feed during the night, allowing you to sleep through. However, in reality few partners actually share the night feeds, so don't be tempted to stop breastfeeding for this reason. There might be an odd occasion when this happens but the novelty wears off very quickly, leaving you firmly back in charge of the night-time feed. This is particularly true when your partner has to get up for work.

Breastfeeding is quite hypnotic and results in the release of endorphin-like substances which help you to settle back to sleep much more quickly, plus you don't have to make up a feed in the middle of the night when your baby is screaming with hunger.

So, what can your partner do to help and support you?

Practical help

If you have other children your partner can take a major practical role in assisting with their care, perhaps helping with the evening and bedtime routines. Fathers who are involved with their children from an early age (such as bathing etc.) tend to be closer to them as they grow older, so encourage him to take a hand in looking after other children while you concentrate on the newest addition.

Emotional help

Your partner needs to be sensitive to your mood changes, particularly in the first few weeks as your body adapts to its new role and your hormones settle. He needs to appreciate that you will be focusing on your new baby's needs and not feel left out. Your relationship changes as you both adapt to the change in your family.

Supporting your independence

Your partner can be a great help in giving you some time to still 'be you'; whether that means taking time to go to the hairdressers, have a massage treatment, go for a gym session or visit a friend, on your own. If your partner is willing and able to look after your new baby then you are likely to feel more relaxed and comfortable about being away from him for a time.

Planning ahead

Before your baby is born you and your partner need to discuss how you would want to deal with a baby who cries constantly or won't sleep. If you can agree in advance on how you will attempt to deal with this it can help you to support each other if things become a little more challenging.

Getting involved

After the first few months, during which you and your baby have worked mainly as a duo (just the two of you spending a lot of time together and baby being largely dependant on you), the relationship becomes a triad, with three people in the group as the father becomes more involved. Once your baby is starting to show his personality, Dad tends to be happy to entertain him for a while, giving you some much-needed 'me' time. Perhaps he would be happy to take over the bath-time routine or lead the run-up to bedtime, getting baby ready for bed, reading a story or playing gently (it is worthwhile suggesting to him that a rough and tumble game before bedtime may be a little too stimulating!).

Friends

Old friends

This is a time when you need your good friends, and soon find out who they are. They will come around, make you a cup of tea, take the baby from you and give you some time to go off and have your shower, walk the dog or do your hair! Anything that just lets you have a little quiet time at some point in the day is a bonus.

As your baby grows, any friends you have, especially with babies of a similar age to yours, are very useful. Your baby will be fascinated by watching others and you will have similar-minded mothers to talk to. As a new mum, your baby is a fascinating subject and all the changes that happen to him are worthy of discussion – other new mums will understand this. A network of friends like this can help to soothe many worries you may have as you realize that something your baby does is actually quite normal and nothing to worry about.

However, do not be tempted to compare everything your baby does with another, as all babies are different. They will all start to walk, talk and smile when they are ready, so try not to let it become something of a competition. It doesn't matter when your baby reaches these milestones, as long as he is happy and healthy – he will get there when he is ready. Your health visitor or doctor will check on him at regular intervals to make sure of this.

You may find that friends without babies tend to have less in common with you at this time, but don't let them go completely. They may be very happy to take the chance of looking after a baby once in a while, giving you a break. And sometimes it is nice to talk 'grown-up' talk with old friends.

It is hoped that you will feel quite comfortable breastfeeding in front of your best friends. They can also help to support your decision to breastfeed in public, so when you have a 'girls' day out' and meet for lunch or coffee, you may feel protected by them as you breastfeed in public. They will be prepared to deal with anyone who challenges, or attempts to prevent, you feeding, but also they can help camouflage you while you are breastfeeding.

Networking

Making friends with a group, perhaps some mothers you met while you were pregnant, maybe at antenatal classes or clinic, can be useful for support. You may wish to get in touch with a local National Childbirth Trust group, La Leche League or similar organization (see below).

When you attend your local clinic to have your baby weighed you may notice the same faces time after time, so you could develop your own local support group. Such a group may already be up and running – ask your midwife or health visitor if they can give you some information. Don't feel you have to attend every single week if you don't want to, but see it as a group of friends rather than a compulsory activity. Your local community centre or church hall may also offer some mother/baby activities. If you were working prior to having your baby, it can be difficult to have a ready-made network of friends, so look out for these opportunities. However, don't be too worried if you feel differently to some of the other mothers you meet – you are an individual, as is your baby. You know what it best for both of you!

Voluntary societies/groups

If you can contact a local support group, such as the National Childbirth Trust or La Leche League, this can give you 'a friend at the end of the phone' when you hit a problem. Often they hold regular meetings where you have the chance to meet up with other mothers who will share their experiences with you to help you overcome your difficulties. You will usually find at least one of these organizations somewhere local to you and it doesn't matter if you didn't attend antenatally, they can be just as helpful once you have had your baby. Details of how to find a local group can be found in 'Taking it further'.

Health professionals

Your midwife will be able to support you fully both in your decision to breastfeed and in giving you advice and practical help to ensure you are successful in breastfeeding. She will be able to answer any questions and help you deal with any problems you may have. Throughout your pregnancy you will see your midwife regularly, so you will have the opportunity to ask her questions in order to prepare yourself. Once you have given birth your midwife will visit you at home to ensure that you and your baby are recovering from the delivery. During this time she will discuss your breastfeeding and be happy to advise you on how to solve any problems you may be having.

A health visitor will take over your care following on from your midwife. She will follow your child's development throughout his early years. This will involve giving advice on feeding, including introduction to solid food, as well as other aspects of health, such as vaccinations.

Being Mum – Jane's experience

Jane was a full-time secretary in an office prior to John's birth. She does hope to go back to work but, for now, wants to stay at home with him. She lives some distance from her own mother and, although she gets on with her partner's parents, they also live active lives.

When John was born, she had a number of visits from friends and family, but now the excitement has died down. Old friends and colleagues are mostly working during the week and it is too far to go to see her mum regularly, but Jane feels she needs some company. She feels a little guilty about this, as she thinks that, perhaps she should be happy to 'stay at home and look after John'.

This is a common problem. New babies are not really very good company. It is likely that, if Jane's breastfeeding has settled and become more established into a routine, a pattern can be seen to her day. So, once the morning routine is over, it may seem a long afternoon, waiting for her partner to come home, by which time she may be so desperate to talk to someone that she 'downloads' her whole day as soon as he walks through the door. At this point he is probably not able to respond the way she would like and so her whole evening starts off badly.

Jane could consider changing her afternoon routine, perhaps meeting up with some of the other mothers she knew during her pregnancy: she could organize a meeting at her own home; they could swap 'birth' stories, and describe how each of their babies is changing. As time goes on, they will have more and more in common, and they can talk about their little worries and concerns. Often these 'problems' can then be seen in perspective and the mother will realize there was really nothing to worry about at all.

Jane could go to an already established group, such as National Childbirth Trust/La Leche League or a local breastfeeding group (some areas have their own Breastfeeding Buddies, or a Breastfeeding Café for example). She could ask her midwife or health visitor if there are any such groups in her area. She could also ask at her local church or community centre; there may be a local mother and toddler or similar group where she could meet other mothers with young children. These may not be breastfeeding-specific, but will still give her the chance to meet up with other new mothers. She could ask her midwife or health visitor if there is a children's centre local to her – there are an increasing number being set up around the country. These provide a number of different services within an area, and she may be able to access breastfeeding support from professionals or groups who meet there.

When Jane takes her baby to see the health visitor she will also have the opportunity to see other new mothers and babies, perhaps at similar ages to John; this may give her another potential group of friends.

Jane could try to plan an event each week. This does not have to be something major – it could just be meeting a friend or going to a 'group' meeting. Once John has gained good head control (usually around five months of age) she could take him swimming. She should aim to get out every day – even just a trip to the shops or a walk round her local area. She will feel more refreshed after getting out for even just a short time.

Practical help

Remember, Supermum does not exist! If anyone offers any help at all, don't say no because you feel guilty, just accept gratefully. You don't have to put any pressure on yourself to get everything done. It is not worth it; you will simply end up not enjoying your baby and the special time you have together.

If possible, enlist some help for the first few weeks. If your partner or another relative (mother, sister, mother-in-law) can be at home with you for the first couple of weeks that is fabulous. Even better is if your partner can have some time off to spend with you and then a relative is around to help once he has gone back to work. Do not try to play hostess though – take advantage of the situation to get some rest while you can. Perhaps your mum would happily vacuum the house, or do the washing and ironing while you rest.

Think about your priorities – what really has to be done. Do not try to cram in all the cleaning and household chores. Make a list of what you really need to do and when. Then you can realistically see what has to be done, as well as how long it might take and what needs to be done first. This will also give you some goals and you can plan around these, including when would be the best time to tackle some of those little jobs.

Think of easy options – if you are cooking meals, double up the amount and freeze some. This will mean you have a second meal ready for a day when things take a little longer than expected. Don't be too concerned about using some little cooking 'cheats' every now and then. Even some of the best cooks do!

Get ahead of yourself. When your baby is down for the night, or if your partner is able to help you with the bedtime routine, take a little time to plan for tomorrow. Restock your changing bag, getting it ready to go for your next trip out.

Expect the unexpected – even the best-laid plans may go awry. Just as you are ready to go out, a dirty nappy or a regurgitated feed may disrupt your plans, so try and build in a little extra time or try not to get too tied to the clock. This can be difficult if you have been very organized prior to the birth of your baby, but try to relax and enjoy motherhood.

Remember to take time to enjoy your new role and make the most of your baby. If you have to go back to work this time can be extra special, so enjoy it and try not to do everything in one day. It really can wait!

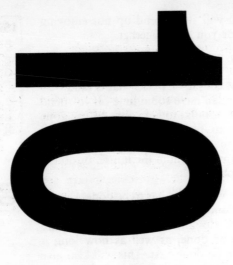

10

introducing solid food to your baby's diet

In this chapter you will learn:
- the best time to start weaning
- how to introduce 'baby-led' weaning
- the best finger foods for your baby
- what foods to avoid.

When to start

Q. When should I start introducing my baby to solids?

It is recommended that your baby should receive breast milk for at least his first six months. You can continue to breastfeed for longer than six months, but at some point after six months your baby will be ready for the introduction of mixed feeding.

Weaning is the introduction of any non-milk foods, in the form of solids, and can also be known as mixed feeding. Weaning does not mean that you have to stop breastfeeding; in fact, you should try to introduce a gradual replacement of breastfeeds. Even if you are bottle-feeding, it is still better not to introduce solids until after six months if you can.

Q. When should I stop breastfeeding?

Many mothers continue to breastfeed for some feeds (or part of feeds), up to the end of the first year and longer, even up to two years. You can continue to breastfeed as well as giving solids to your baby. Do not feel under too much pressure to introduce mixed feeding too early; it can sometimes feel a bit like a competition and you may feel you are constantly being questioned or criticized because you are still breastfeeding your baby. Try to ignore others – if you and your baby are still happy with breastfeeding, then carry on.

Introducing new foods gradually helps your baby to adjust to new tastes, but also ensures you do not reduce your milk supply suddenly. Remember that once you do start to introduce foods other than breast milk your baby's bowel habits will change. They will no longer be yellow and sweet smelling but become firmer, darker and smellier.

Advice regarding when to start weaning has changed considerably over the years, so if you talk to your relatives and friends it can be quite confusing to actually know what is best for your baby. It used to be normal to commence weaning at around three months; this then moved towards four months; then four to six months; and now from six months onwards. The advice given now about how to introduce food to a six-month-old has not really changed from when discussing weaning for a three-month-old; however, really this should be quite different as a six-month-old has far more skills than a three-month-old.

Three-month-old babies are really only used to liquids, so traditionally this baby was given purées which became increasingly thicker or consisted of mashed foods, before finally he was able to take more lumpy foods. At this age the baby is sucking the mixture off the spoon, which means it goes straight to the back of the mouth and may cause him to 'gag'. However, a six-month-old does not really need to go through the stages of puréed and mashed foods.

Q. How much food should I give my baby?

A new approach to weaning is 'baby-led' weaning, which allows the baby to progress on to solids when he is ready and at his own pace. Baby-led weaning is thought to be more appropriate for babies of six months and older as they can control what and how much they take. This follows on from baby-led breastfeeding and is particularly suited to the breastfed infant because as and when your baby develops the appropriate skills he will be ready to start exploring solids.

It is suggested that feeding (milk) and starting solids should be separated. This enables your baby to explore taking solid food out of curiosity rather than hunger. This can mean a more relaxed approach towards solids as they are not seen as a necessity for feeding. If your baby then requires a breastfeed he will naturally adjust the amount and length of the feed in response to his appetite, so you don't have to make a decision about when to stop or cut-down. As your baby joins in family mealtimes and eats more 'solid' food he will reduce the amount of breast milk he asks for.

This will be different for babies who have been formula fed as the consistency and constituents of the milk feed do not change as breast milk does, and your baby may need to be offered water as a drink with his food in order to avoid consuming too many calories or too few. You may need to discuss this method of weaning with your health visitor.

At six months old your baby will be used to sitting up watching you (if supported), his neck muscles will be strong enough to support his head and he will have good hand–eye coordination so he is now able to reach out, grasp anything you put in his hand and put it to his mouth. At this age also, your baby will try to imitate you, so when he sees you eating and chewing, he will attempt to 'chew' and move his jaw and mouth accordingly.

One of the differences your baby has to adjust to when you start weaning is the fact that his meal is no longer in one continuous flow. He also has to learn to move food to the back of the throat, ready for swallowing. Babies seem to learn how to move their food towards the back of their mouths once they have learnt to chew. Similarly, they develop the ability to chew after they have developed the ability to reach out and grab objects. They are unable to pick up small items at this stage. So it seems to make sense that young babies are not able to put themselves at risk by putting small pieces of foods into their mouths because they have not developed the skills to pick up small pieces before they have developed the ability to chew.

Throughout the time you are introducing solid foods to your baby, you can continue to breastfeed. The amount of breast milk your baby will take will drop as the amounts of solid foods increase. Ultimately, your baby will reach a point when the only breastfeed he has will be at bedtime, or during the night. If your baby is ill, you might notice he doesn't want to eat as normal, and at such times you may find he will increase his demand for breast milk. This will help to maintain his intake and keep him hydrated while he recovers.

How to start introducing solids

It is a good idea, initially, to introduce just one foodstuff at a time; this will let you see its effect on your baby. If you know there is a history of food allergy in the family it is probably best to avoid particular foods, which are most linked with allergies, until later as your baby may also be sensitive to these foods. If you do decide to introduce some solids prior to six months then it is best to avoid wheat, gluten, fish, shellfish, eggs, liver, citrus foods, and soft or unpasteurized cheeses.

If you have left weaning until your baby is six months old, you may still wish to introduce mashed foods first, especially if your baby has been bottle-feeding. Then introduce finger foods as soon as your baby is ready; for some babies this may be almost right away.

When introducing mashed or puréed foods, it is best to start with fruit or vegetable purées, usually giving just one or two teaspoons following a breastfeed or in the middle of a feed. This should mean that your baby is not too hungry and will be more prepared to try mixed foods.

Try to choose a time of the day when you are less hurried or your baby may pick up on your cues and feel anxious. Do not be tempted to give your baby only foods you like, avoiding others you dislike. Give him a wide variety of tastes, including those you don't like, as he may like them. Don't be in a rush to hurry this process; your breast milk is a good basis for mixed feeding. While your baby is adjusting to taking solids, he can continue with your breast milk for as long as necessary.

You should continue to give your baby milk until he is at least 12 months of age; he is likely still to need around 500 ml to 600 ml (about a pint) of milk each day. Ideally you should use breast milk, although formula milk is also an option; you should not give normal cows' milk, goats' milk, sheep's milk, oat-based milk or rice-based milk to your baby at this age as these options do not contain enough nutrients. An alternative drink could be water (before the age of six months this should be previously boiled and cooled), but if you wish to give your baby juice to drink this should be diluted, one part juice to ten parts water.

How to encourage 'baby-led' weaning

Baby-led weaning is a natural progression from breastfeeding your baby. It allows him to proceed at his own pace. You will know when your baby is ready as he will be able to sit up, show interest in solid foods, may pick up food and put it in his mouth, seems to try to chew and may have teeth, and may seem hungry despite having increased milk feeds for several days. Do not be tempted to add anything to a bottle, such as baby rice or rusk, in order to satisfy his hunger. If he is still hungry, is over six months of age and you have tried increasing milk feeds which have not helped, then it may be time to consider mixed feeding.

Your baby will be able to sample a variety of foods, testing out a range of textures, tastes and shapes. This will allow your baby to try out a range of different foods and leave what he doesn't like, rather than rejecting a whole 'meal' beacause it contains something he doesn't want.

Food should be prepared in 'baby-fist' sizes – chunks (chip-shaped) rather than smaller bite-sized pieces, or foods with stalks which enable the baby to hold them more easily. Your baby can then hold the food in his fist and suck on it until it is softened and he can then chew it. Your baby does not need teeth to chew; his gums will be perfectly adequate. Obviously harder foods, such as carrots and other vegetables, will need to be cooked first to soften them. Do not give him small round pieces of food, such as grapes, without cutting them in half first. If giving your baby meat, it is best to give this in one larger piece so he can suck on it until it is softened and ready to chew. When starting to feed your baby never leave him alone, to ensure he doesn't choke; talk to him, gently encouraging him. Do not try to give him solids if he seems disinterested, is frustrated or upset, or if he seems unwell or not himself.

Ensure that your baby is sitting upright in a chair, facing forward, safely secured – this will allow him to explore feeding himself with his fingers. Let him touch and feel his food. You could give your baby a spoon and let him experiment with feeding himself – it will be messy (so cover the floor and yourselves) but this way he learns new skills and leads the way, stopping when he has had enough, just as he has done while breastfeeding.

When preparing foods for your baby, do not add salt or sugar to your cooking. Remember that some foods naturally contain salt, such as bacon and some cheese, so be careful if using such products. Initially, mashed vegetables can be introduced, such as carrots, parsnips, potatoes, yams, bananas, avocado, cooked apples or pears. Cook foods until soft and then cut them into finger-sized pieces if your baby seems interested. Let your baby have as much food as he wants – don't worry that he is not taking very much. Initially he just needs to get used to taking foods other than milk. When he loses interest, turns away, won't open his mouth or pushes food away your baby is telling you he doesn't want any more. It may not seem that he has had very much, but the amount will increase.

Make the experience pleasant; sit with your baby, chatting to him, getting him to try a range of different tastes and textures; stop trying to get him to eat the food when it is refused.

Try to avoid giving your baby sweet biscuits or rusks as he may develop a sweet tooth. Do not give honey to your baby until he is at least a year old as it can contain a type of bacteria that produce toxins which can make him very ill.

If you prefer not to give your baby meat, then you should make sure that he receives pulses, tofu, soya or eggs in order to ensure a sufficient intake of protein.

What foods to avoid

Avoid giving your baby the following:

- Salt – do not add this to your cooking or when preparing food for your baby. Babies' kidneys cannot tolerate too much salt.
- Sugar – this should be avoided as it can lead to a sweet tooth and tooth decay when the teeth come in.
- Honey – this should not be added to foods given to children under the age of one year as it can contain bacteria that produce a toxin which can lead to a serious condition called botulism.
- Nuts – these are a potential choking hazard for young children under the age of five years, as well as being a potential allergen.
- Low-fat foods – low-fat fromage frais, yoghurts and other dairy producs are not suitable for children under the age of two. Important calories and energy is sourced from fat and this is essential in a child's diet.

As your baby continues to develop you can introduce other foods, such as eggs (well cooked until the white and yolk are solid) or small pieces of meat or chicken. And as he increases the amount of mixed food he takes, you will find he takes less breast milk. You can start to offer your baby a drink of water with food if he is over six months of age; this can be directly from the tap, it does not have to be boiled and cooled (although this should still be done if you are preparing formula milk). There is no reason to use bottled water as this can contain other concentrated minerals that are unnecessary. If you are giving him formula milk you may find you can drop a feed, although you should continue giving formula milk until he is at least 12 months of age.

Your baby requires adequate amounts of vitamin D among other nutrients; this is only found in a small number of foods such as fortified margarine, eggs and fatty fish. It is also made by the body as a result of being exposed to sunlight, although this should only be gentle sunlight as exposure to strong sunlight is not encouraged due its adverse effects. Therefore all children between the ages of one and five years should receive vitamin drops.

Babies use a lot of energy, and this is provided by fat in the diet. Babies need full-fat foods in their diet in order to meet their energy requirements. It is not recommended that babies under the age of two are given low-fat foods, even if other family members may be on low-fat diets, as they will not gain sufficient nutritional benefits. Children over two years old who eat well can have semi-skimmed milk if you prefer, but those under five should not be given skimmed milk.

Finger foods to try

- Toast or pitta bread
- Cooked pasta shapes
- Lightly cooked vegetables, such as carrots, green beans, cauliflower, broccoli
- Soft, ripe, peeled fruits; melon, banana, pear, peach
- Cooked apple
- Small cubes or slices of cheese.

Home-made or ready-prepared food?

When you first introduce mixed feeding for your baby it may seem rather time-consuming to prepare such small amounts of food, especially when he may then not appear to be very fond of it. It can be quite tempting and convenient to try ready-prepared food, as this can be kept in a sealed container for subsequent meals. Also, if you prepare the food yourself and baby does not want it you can often feel you have wasted your time and feel rejected or hurt that your baby doesn't seem to like it. Do not be put off though; give it to him again at a later time as he may be happy to try it then. It can be quite costly to buy ready-prepared jars or cans of baby food but you can divide it for use at more than one mealtime, although you should not keep food already offered to your baby and left over.

When preparing the family meal, keep some of this and store or freeze it so you don't have to then cook something especially for your baby. For example, when cooking the vegetables, put some of these to one side prior to adding any salt or seasoning. They can be used as finger food or mashed and given to your baby that way. This will make it easier to include your baby in family mealtimes and he will learn to eat the same foods. However, when preparing family meals do also check the labels of any ingredients to ensure they are not high in salt or sugar.

If you decide to use ready-prepared foods, either as an alternative occasionally or more regularly, you will need to read the labels carefully. Make sure the products are suitable for the age of your baby, and do not contain foods that should be avoided by young babies. They are generally labelled as Stage 1, 2 or 3. Stage 1 is around six months and you should aim to introduce your baby to a range of various foods; stage 2 is six to nine months and is when your baby is taking three meals per day; and stage 3 is over one year of age. You should also ensure that the product has not date-expired; check the 'use by' and 'best-before' dates. Check that the seals are not broken to ensure containers have not been previously opened.

Try to avoid giving tea, coffee or caffeinated drinks as these can prevent the absorption of iron. Iron stores are laid down during pregnancy and are enough to last your baby until he is six months old. When you introduce mixed feeding this can help supplement the iron status of your baby. Iron is found in meat and fish, but also in plants such as cereals, dark green vegetables and dried fruits.

If you feed your baby meat, it is helpful to serve this together with vegetables or pulses as these can aid the absorption of the iron in the meat. Vitamin C also helps in the absorption of iron from non-meat sources, as discussed when talking about the constituents of breast milk (see Chapter 02).

Once your baby is taking several meals each day he will also need snacks during the day. He still only has a small stomach and gets full quite quickly, so he will need snacks to maintain his energy levels. Make sure these are healthy, not high in sugar or salt content. Ideal snack foods include breadsticks, a cracker with a little cheese, slices of banana, small portions of (full-fat) fromage frais or yoghurt.

Teach your baby good habits – washing his hands before eating, for example. This will then become a habit that, it is hoped, will continue through your child's life. Try to introduce a cup/beaker rather than a bottle with meals, especially if you have been breastfeeding. It is suggested that you try to introduce a cup in place of a bottle once your baby reaches the age of one year, as sucking from a bottle teat can lead to speech delay and damage the teeth, particularly if drinking sweetened drinks. Habits and tastes developed at this stage are likely to continue into childhood and later life.

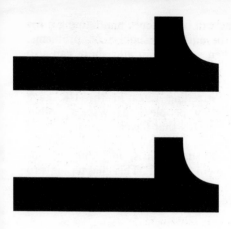

11

breastfeeding and society

In this chapter you will learn:

- about the Baby Friendly Initiative
- how Baby Friendly can help support breastfeeding
- about breastfeeding in public
- about your right to breastfeed in public
- about going on holiday with your breastfed baby.

Just as starting breastfeeding can be difficult, maintaining it for as long as you want can be equally fraught with problems. Breastfeeding your baby when you are out and about can also be quite a challenge. This is not really helped by the fact that breastfeeding is not really seen as part of British culture. Over the last few decades, breastfeeding rates in the UK have declined, with the result that few people actually see a mother breastfeeding her baby. This means that fewer women will feel comfortable about breastfeeding their baby in public. Bottle-feeding is seen on an almost daily basis, including in our favourite 'soaps', making it seem 'normal'. This chapter aims to give you some information to help support you in feeling comfortable about breastfeeding as part of your daily life.

What is the Baby Friendly Initiative?

The Baby Friendly Initiative (BFI) was launched in 1991 jointly by UNICEF and the World Health Organization (WHO). It aims to promote and support breastfeeding. It came about because many women who wished to breastfeed were giving up within the first four to six weeks. It identified some of the reasons many women were giving up breastfeeding, including receiving conflicting advice when they were in hospital, and feeling unsupported while breastfeeding. This project intended to try to ensure that all health professionals were giving the same information to women so they could decide how to feed their baby and knew how to overcome any problems they might experience.

A project was launched to get local groups together to look at local policies, review the education health professionals receive and generally raise awareness of the benefits of breastfeeding. As a result of this work a global initiative was developed to promote 'Baby Friendly' hospitals. This is an award maternity units can apply for to demonstrate that they are committed to supporting breastfeeding. To gain a 'Baby Friendly' award the hospital is independently assessed against a set of ten criteria (Ten Steps). If your local maternity unit has gained 'Baby Friendly' status you can be sure it will be committed to supporting your breastfeeding.

Ten Steps to Successful Breastfeeding

In order to achieve Baby Friendly status, every facility providing maternity services and care for newborn infants in the hospital should:

1 Have a written breastfeeding policy that is routinely communicated to all healthcare staff.
2 Train all health care staff in the skills necessary to implement the breastfeeding policy.
3 Inform all pregnant women about the benefits and management of breastfeeding.
4 Help mothers to initiate breastfeeding within half an hour of giving birth.
5 Show mothers how to breastfeed and how to maintain lactation even if they are separated from their infants.
6 Give newborn infants no food or drink other than breast milk, unless medically indicated.
7 Practise rooming-in, allowing mothers and infants to remain together for 24 hours a day.
8 Encourage breastfeeding on demand.
9 Give no artificial teats or pacifiers (also called dummies or soothers) to breastfeeding infants.
10 Foster the establishment of breastfeeding support groups and refer mothers to them on discharge from hospital or clinic.

Q. Is it just for hospitals?

Although this project was initially focused on hospitals, it was soon recognized that in the United Kingdom women spend very little time in hospital compared with women in other countries, so the initiative has been extended into community settings as a Seven-Point Plan. This is based on the Ten Steps used for hospitals, and a number of healthcare trusts and facilities now carry a BFI certificate of commitment or accreditation.

Seven-Point Plan for the Protection, Promotion and Support of Breastfeeding in Community Healthcare Settings

In order to achieve Baby Friendly status, the healthcare setting should:

1 Have a written breastfeeding policy that is routinely communicated to all healthcare staff.

2 Train all healthcare staff involved in the care of mothers and babies in the skills necessary to implement the policy.

3 Inform all pregnant women about the benefits and management of breastfeeding.

4 Support mothers to initiate and maintain breastfeeding.

5 Encourage exclusive and continued breastfeeding, with appropriately timed introduction of complementary foods.

6 Provide a welcoming atmosphere for breastfeeding families.

7 Promote cooperation between healthcare staff, community support groups and the local community.

What does it mean for you?

If you have your baby in a Baby Friendly accredited maternity unit you know that all the health professionals you meet will offer you the highest standards of care and follow best practice in relation to breastfeeding. While you are pregnant you will be given information about feeding your baby, including information about the benefits of breastfeeding. This will allow you to make a fully informed choice about how you want to feed your baby. You can expect to experience skin-to-skin contact and hold your baby straight after delivery. If you do decide to breastfeed you will receive help to put your baby to the breast within half an hour of delivery, clear consistent advice on how to breastfeed, as well as help to position your baby and help him to 'latch on'. A midwife will help you with this and no bottles or artificial milk will be offered to your baby unless there is a valid medical reason for this. Your baby will stay with you all the time – known as 'rooming- in'.

Q. How many maternity units are 'Baby Friendly'?

Up to May 2008 there were 53 maternity hospitals in the UK with full accreditation, while a further 89 were in the process of working towards becoming 'Baby Friendly', with either a Certificate of Commitment or undergoing the various stages for full approval and accreditation. You can find out if your local maternity hospital is among these by visiting the Baby Friendly Initiative website at www.babyfriendly.org.uk and looking under 'Awards'.

All of the UK is listed on the Baby Friendly Initiative website. Some parts of the country do a lot better than others. In particular, more births take place in a Baby Friendly unit in Scotland than anywhere else in the UK, while England has the lowest percentage. However, this does vary vastly throughout England, with many parts of London and the South-East coming off worst with 0% of births taking place in a Baby Friendly hospital, while if you live in the County Durham and Tees Valley area there are over 37% of births in a Baby Friendly unit. These figures will change regularly as more units undergo the stringent process leading to full accreditation. There have been strong recommendations made to try and ensure all maternity units work towards these principles.

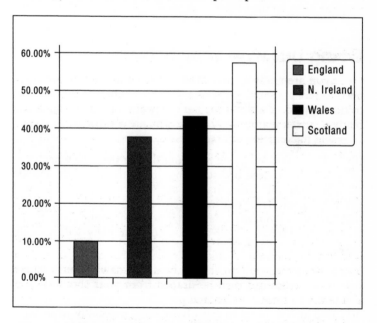

figure 11.1 Bar chart showing percentage of babies born in Baby Friendly hospitals (**www.babyfriendly.org.uk**)

Q. What if I don't want to breastfeed – will I have to if my local unit is 'Baby Friendly'?

If you decide that breastfeeding is not for you, you will still receive help and support to feed your baby safely, for example in making up a bottle. Staff will be able to answer any questions you might have. The decision is yours; it is your baby and you decide. Obviously the staff will give you all the information to help you in this decision, but be honest – if you want to bottle-feed don't be afraid to say so. Don't feel you have to breastfeed just because someone might expect you to. Breastfeed because you want to – there are lots of good reasons to – but you must decide that *you* want to, otherwise you may feel resentful at having to try when your midwife could instead be using that time to discuss with you the principles of safely bottle-feeding. But don't be too ready to dismiss it either; be prepared to listen to the advice and information you will be offered while you are pregnant and you may find yourself changing your mind from being a determined bottle-feeder to actually wanting to try to put your baby to the breast.

Going out with your baby

Once you are ready to take your baby out and about, you will need to feel prepared for your excursions, whether this is a trip to the shops or a walk to the park. Always have a changing bag ready – repack it after every trip so you are always 'ready to go'. This will make going out seem less daunting.

If you know you are going to be out during the time when your baby is likely to need breastfeeding, think ahead a little. Decide on what you will wear, making sure it is something that will easily accommodate your little breast-feeder – perhaps a blouse that can open from the side or that you can unbutton from the bottom in order to lift up slightly so your baby will actually cover up most of your breast when feeding.

You may find it useful to carry a blanket, shawl or terry nappy with you. These can then be draped from your shoulder over your baby to form a screen and protect your privacy more. You may find also it useful to use a baby sling, especially while your baby is smaller. This can allow you to carry your baby while keeping your arms free, but will also allow for very discrete feeding.

If you are shopping with your baby, you will get to know the best places for breastfeeding. Some shopping centres have specific areas set aside for breastfeeding mothers; or there may be very good facilities in a particular shop where you will feel comfortable while breastfeeding.

Up until recently breastfeeding mothers in England did not have the right to breastfeed in public; however, plans were announced in June 2008 that will give legal support for women to breastfeed their young babies. Women in Scotland have had the legal right to breastfeed their babies in public since 2005.

Essentials for the changing bag

- Think about the size when buying your bag and consider what type you want, e.g. shoulder bag or backpack.

- Choose a washable material, but moisture resistant, so it can be wiped down as necessary.

- Some changing bags have detachable 'mats' so wherever you are you have something on which to lay your baby.

- Storage pockets are useful; the more the better usually. Make sure the pockets are of a useful size to fit the items you want to take.

- Keep your bag topped up with nappies, disposable nappy bags, some bottom wipes as well as some cotton wool. This way, if you have access to water you can use it; if not then use the baby wipes. It won't hurt occasionally.

- Put in a change of clothes also, just in case of accidents.

Breastfeeding in public

However confident you feel, when it comes to breastfeeding your baby in public, this can be quite daunting. The worry of being 'thrown out' of a restaurant will, no doubt, be in your thoughts. There is always the fear that you may upset someone while giving your baby his lunch, which can be quite intimidating; young people may look at you with disgust, older people may pass by you 'tutt-tutting', businesswomen may stare at you pointedly. Sometimes it can feel as if you are taking on the whole world. However, it is becoming more accepted and more and more places are providing suitable accommodation where you can comfortably breastfeed your baby.

Feeding when out with baby – Emma's experience

Emma is concerned about feeding her baby, Rosie, when going out, especially if she is shopping. She now feels able to latch Rosie on quite quickly and competently, but she is worried in case someone feels offended by her breastfeeding, especially if this might result in her being asked to move or stop feeding. Emma feels that she should not be expected to feed in a toilet but equally does not intend to deliberately upset anyone else.

Emma's choice of clothing when going out is worth thinking about, as some blouses or tops will allow for more discrete feeding. Wearing a pashmina over her shoulder while feeding will also allow for greater privacy.

Emma should also watch for hunger cues from Rosie and start breastfeeding as soon as she can rather than waiting for Rosie to be desperate for a feed. This will mean that Rosie isn't crying frantically, which itself will attract attention, and she will go to the breast more easily than when she is too 'worked up'.

If intending to breastfeed in a restaurant or café, Emma could try to find a table in a booth, or at least near a wall. This way she will be able to turn away while attaching Rosie at the breast and then turn back when she is happily suckling. She may notice more mothers sitting in certain areas; this could be a good indicator that it is a good area for her to breastfeed.

If attending any local network or breastfeeding groups, other breastfeeding mothers may be able to tell Emma some of the best places to feed. The National Childbirth Trust often undertakes surveys to identify the best restaurants/cafes in an area, so ask she could ask her local NCT group for advice too.

Emma's might like to practise feeding before she makes the move to feed in public. She could ask a friend or her partner to look at her while she is feeding, or watch herself in a mirror; this way she will see how 'invisible' breastfeeding can be.

If Emma really feels too embarrassed to breastfeed, especially if out on her own, then it might be possible to breastfeed in the car (if she has one) before starting, or retreat to the car when necessary. This is not such a good idea if it is a hot day though.

Clothes tips

- Look through your wardrobe to identify the tops that will give easiest access to your breast.
- You could wear a vest top underneath a wraparound, or a cardigan which can then be pulled together once baby is well positioned.
- There are a number of companies that sell 'specific' breastfeeding-friendly clothing; these are worth considering if your budget runs to it, but do look into how you could wear and adapt your current wardrobe.
- Don't forget to consider which bras would also be easiest to open one-handed; perhaps one with an under-cup zipper.
- Practise using different clothing and bras whenever you feed your baby, to determine which you find best.

Travelling

Going abroad with a breastfeeding baby is relatively easy. You don't have to worry whether to take sufficient supplies of his 'favourite' food or regular milk supply in case you can't find it locally. Also, nappies etc. can usually be found abroad, so think carefully about what you really need to take with you. You also need to consider your travelling arrangements; are you driving (via tunnel or ferry), going by train or flying?

Flying

If you are flying, depending upon your baby's age, you may have to share your seat with him on your lap – children under the age of two do not have their own seat. However, when booking your flight try to reserve a 'front' (bulk-head) seat; this gives you more room and often an in-flight cot can be provided (probably best to ask for this when booking). It may be worth asking when you check in at the airport if they could leave the seat next to you empty, unless absolutely necessary. It is possible to purchase specific child safety straps if your baby is going to have a seat of his own.

You will usually have to have your baby on your lap for take off and landing, so during these times, breastfeed him. This will help equalize the pressure in his ears as he is too young to be able to yawn or swallow to make his ears 'pop'. You will need to start feeding him as soon as the descent begins and continue until it has finished. If he is slightly older and taking water or juice, you could give him this instead; he just needs to keep swallowing.

Don't give him any medication to help him sleep; this often has the opposite effect. Take a cosy blanket as the temperature can drop once in flight. The air within an aircraft is recycled so can be quite dry, which may make your baby a little irritated or 'snuffly'. A damp cloth to wipe his face every now and then can help to relieve this a little. Difficult as it may be, try not to worry too much how other passengers may react to your baby – that is their problem. Don't feel the need to apologize for him being there. Obviously take things with you to keep him amused but if you are stressed your baby will pick up on this and react accordingly.

Changing your baby can be a little challenging on board an aircraft. Check which toilets have changing facilities; sometimes this is restricted to the rear of plane. Try to change your baby as close to boarding as possible, although this will not always mean that you do not need to change him as soon as you have got on board!

Driving

Having your own transport can mean that you don't need to worry about what you take with you. However, it is not a good idea to breastfeed while the car is being driven. Your baby should be securely fastened into a car seat throughout the journey. If you do decide to breastfeed, it is safer to wait until the car can pull over and stop before removing him from his seat to feed.

If you are travelling from the UK to Europe you might be able to sit comfortably in your car while going through the Channel Tunnel, for example, so your baby is not disturbed and may sleep throughout the train journey. Even if he wakes you may find it easier to cope without having to worry about disturbing other passengers.

Your journey may include taking your car on a ferry. If so you will have the freedom to walk around for the entire journey, finding a host of things with which to amuse your baby. You may wish to book a cabin for the journey to give you somewhere to rest and breastfeed if it is a longer crossing, especially overnight.

Travelling by train

Travelling abroad by train from the UK will usually mean taking Eurostar. Children under the age of four usually travel free and you can ask for seats in the family area, which is also close to the changing facilities. This will mean there is a lot for your baby to see and help keep him occupied. The seating is around a table so there is somewhere for you to put everything. You can get up and walk around and be free to amuse your baby. On some longer journeys the train may have bunk beds and couchettes, which can give you some privacy and space in which to rest and relax, although space is a little limited.

Breastfeeding abroad

This is usually far more relaxed than in the UK, particularly when in Europe. Many European countries are far more accepting of breastfeeding and of children in general. You are far less likely to encounter any adverse comments, often quite the contrary. You will find there are fewer places for 'changing' your baby, but it is quite accepted for you to breastfeed whenever this is necessary. Take some time to research the country and area you intend to visit; there are some countries where women are expected to keep their bodies covered, and breastfeeding in public may also be unacceptable. The use of a light shawl may be useful for when you do need to feed.

Remember that, depending upon the time of year, many countries are likely to be hotter than the UK, so your baby will probably want to be breastfed more frequently in order to quench his thirst. Adapt to your baby's new routine if you can. You will probably need to drink more yourself too in order to avoid becoming dehydrated, which would reduce your milk supply. Do carry some cleansing wipes with you so you can keep your breasts clean and fresh while travelling.

If you are breastfeeding, it is less likely that your baby will become ill from food poisoning. However, you do need to take care of yourself so you do not become ill as this may affect your milk supply, particularly if you become dehydrated.

In general, travelling abroad with your breastfed baby is relatively hassle-free as you will not have to worry about having somewhere to make up bottles of formula, or finding water to make up the feed. You can just relax and enjoy yourself; try not to be too rigid in your routine but adapt to your baby's needs.

taking it further

Finding help and further information

Throughout this book I have tried to help you find solutions to some of the problems or concerns you may encounter while breastfeeding. Remember that in the early weeks your midwife is there to support you; she will give you her contact details so if you have a problem you will be able to speak to her when you need her most. After the first couple of weeks you will probably be in contact with your health visitor who should also be able to give you advice when you need it.

However, sometimes you may feel that you need more support than this and a number of organizations employ breastfeeding counsellors who have usually been breastfeeding mothers themselves, so are well equipped to help you. A number of these organizations are also able to help you find more information on a number of related issues.

Organization contact details

Where to go for further help
CRY-SIS
www.cry-sis.org.uk
Tel: 08451 228 669

La Leche League (LLL)
P.O. Box 29
West Bridgford
Nottingham
NG2 7NP
www.laleche.org.uk
Helpline: 0845 120 2918

National Childbirth Trust (NCT)
Alexandra House
Oldham Terrace
London
W3 6NH
www.nct.org.uk
Breastfeeding line: 0870 444 8708

TAMBA (Twins and Multiple Births Association)
2 The Willows
Gardner Road
Guildford
GU1 4PG
www.tamba.org.uk
Twinline – support line: 0800 138 0509

MAMA (Meet a Mum Association)
www.mama.co.uk
Helpline: 0845 120 3746 (weekdays only, 7pm–10pm)

Association of Breastfeeding Mothers
www.abm.me.uk
Counselling hotline: 08444 122 949

Further information can be obtained from
Baby Friendly Initiative
www.babyfriendly.org.uk

Breastfeeding Network
P.O. Box 11126
Paisley
PA2 8YB
www.breastfeedingnetwork.org.uk
Supporterline: 0844 412 4664

Department for Business Enterprise and Regulatory Reform
Download document entitled 'Pregnancy and Work – What you
need to know as an employee'
www.berr.gov.uk

Health & Safety Executive (HSE)
www.hse/gov.uk/mothers

The NHS website
Download document entitled 'Breastfeeding and Work –
Information for employees and employers'
www.breastfeeding.nhs.uk

UK Association for Milk Banking
Find information about donating breast milk and milk banking
at
info@ukamb.org
www.ukamb.org
Tel: 020 8383 3559

Baby-led weaning
www.rapleyweaning.com
www.babyledweaning.co.uk

Further reading

La Leche League International (2004) *The Womanly Art of
Breastfeeding*

Lang, Sandra (2002) *Breastfeeding Special Care Babies*

Royal College of Midwives (2002) *Successful Breastfeeding*

index

teach® yourself

From Advanced Sudoku to Zulu, you'll find everything you need in the **teach yourself** range, in books, on CD and on DVD.

Visit **www.teachyourself.co.uk** for more details.

Advanced Sudoku and Kakuro
Afrikaans
Alexander Technique
Algebra
Ancient Greek
Applied Psychology
Arabic
Arabic Conversation
Aromatherapy
Art History
Astrology
Astronomy
AutoCAD 2004
AutoCAD 2007
Ayurveda
Baby Massage and Yoga
Baby Signing
Baby Sleep
Bach Flower Remedies
Backgammon
Ballroom Dancing
Basic Accounting
Basic Computer Skills
Basic Mathematics
Beauty
Beekeeping
Beginner's Arabic Script
Beginner's Chinese Script
Beginner's Dutch

Beginner's French
Beginner's German
Beginner's Greek
Beginner's Greek Script
Beginner's Hindi
Beginner's Hindi Script
Beginner's Italian
Beginner's Japanese
Beginner's Japanese Script
Beginner's Latin
Beginner's Mandarin Chinese
Beginner's Portuguese
Beginner's Russian
Beginner's Russian Script
Beginner's Spanish
Beginner's Turkish
Beginner's Urdu Script
Bengali
Better Bridge
Better Chess
Better Driving
Better Handwriting
Biblical Hebrew
Biology
Birdwatching
Blogging
Body Language
Book Keeping
Brazilian Portuguese

Bridge
British Citizenship Test, The
British Empire, The
British Monarchy from Henry
  VIII, The
Buddhism
Bulgarian
Bulgarian Conversation
Business French
Business Plans
Business Spanish
Business Studies
C++
Calculus
Calligraphy
Cantonese
Caravanning
Car Buying and Maintenance
Card Games
Catalan
Chess
Chi Kung
Chinese Medicine
Christianity
Classical Music
Coaching
Cold War, The
Collecting
Computing for the Over 50s
Consulting
Copywriting
Correct English
Counselling
Creative Writing
Cricket
Croatian
Crystal Healing
CVs
Czech
Danish
Decluttering
Desktop Publishing
Detox
Digital Home Movie Making
Digital Photography
Dog Training
Drawing

Dream Interpretation
Dutch
Dutch Conversation
Dutch Dictionary
Dutch Grammar
Eastern Philosophy
Electronics
English as a Foreign Language
English Grammar
English Grammar as a Foreign
  Language
Entrepreneurship
Estonian
Ethics
Excel 2003
Feng Shui
Film Making
Film Studies
Finance for Non-Financial
  Managers
Finnish
First World War, The
Fitness
Flash 8
Flash MX
Flexible Working
Flirting
Flower Arranging
Franchising
French
French Conversation
French Dictionary
French for Homebuyers
French Grammar
French Phrasebook
French Starter Kit
French Verbs
French Vocabulary
Freud
Gaelic
Gaelic Conversation
Gaelic Dictionary
Gardening
Genetics
Geology
German
German Conversation

Managing Stress
Managing Your Own Career
Mandarin Chinese
Mandarin Chinese Conversation
Marketing
Marx
Massage
Mathematics
Meditation
Middle East Since 1945, The
Modern China
Modern Hebrew
Modern Persian
Mosaics
Music Theory
Mussolini's Italy
Nazi Germany
Negotiating
Nepali
New Testament Greek
NLP
Norwegian
Norwegian Conversation
Old English
One-Day French
One-Day French – the DVD
One-Day German
One-Day Greek
One-Day Italian
One-Day Polish
One-Day Portuguese
One-Day Spanish
One-Day Spanish – the DVD
One-Day Turkish
Origami
Owning a Cat
Owning a Horse
Panjabi
PC Networking for Small
  Businesses
Personal Safety and Self
  Defence
Philosophy
Philosophy of Mind
Philosophy of Religion
Phone French
Phone German

Phone Italian
Phone Japanese
Phone Mandarin Chinese
Phone Spanish
Photography
Photoshop
PHP with MySQL
Physics
Piano
Pilates
Planning Your Wedding
Polish
Polish Conversation
Politics
Portuguese
Portuguese Conversation
Portuguese for Homebuyers
Portuguese Grammar
Portuguese Phrasebook
Postmodernism
Pottery
PowerPoint 2003
PR
Project Management
Psychology
Quick Fix French Grammar
Quick Fix German Grammar
Quick Fix Italian Grammar
Quick Fix Spanish Grammar
Quick Fix: Access 2002
Quick Fix: Excel 2000
Quick Fix: Excel 2002
Quick Fix: HTML
Quick Fix: Windows XP
Quick Fix: Word
Quilting
Recruitment
Reflexology
Reiki
Relaxation
Retaining Staff
Romanian
Running Your Own Business
Russian
Russian Conversation
Russian Grammar
Sage Line 50

Sanskrit
Screenwriting
Second World War, The
Serbian
Setting Up a Small Business
Shorthand Pitman 2000
Sikhism
Singing
Slovene
Small Business Accounting
Small Business Health Check
Songwriting
Spanish
Spanish Conversation
Spanish Dictionary
Spanish for Homebuyers
Spanish Grammar
Spanish Phrasebook
Spanish Starter Kit
Spanish Verbs
Spanish Vocabulary
Speaking On Special Occasions
Speed Reading
Stalin's Russia
Stand Up Comedy
Statistics
Stop Smoking
Sudoku
Swahili
Swahili Dictionary
Swedish
Swedish Conversation
Tagalog
Tai Chi
Tantric Sex
Tap Dancing
Teaching English as a Foreign
    Language
Teams & Team Working
Thai
Thai Conversation
Theatre
Time Management
Tracing Your Family History
Training
Travel Writing
Trigonometry

Turkish
Turkish Conversation
Twentieth Century USA
Typing
Ukrainian
Understanding Tax for Small
    Businesses
Understanding Terrorism
Urdu
Vietnamese
Visual Basic
Volcanoes, Earthquakes and
    Tsunamis
Watercolour Painting
Weight Control through Diet &
    Exercise
Welsh
Welsh Conversation
Welsh Dictionary
Welsh Grammar
Wills & Probate
Windows XP
Wine Tasting
Winning at Job Interviews
Word 2003
World Faiths
Writing Crime Fiction
Writing for Children
Writing for Magazines
Writing a Novel
Writing a Play
Writing Poetry
Xhosa
Yiddish
Yoga
Your Wedding
Zen
Zulu

teach yourself	**feeding your baby** judy more

- Are you tired of 'gurus' and their menu planners?
- Do you want a healthy diet your baby will enjoy?
- Do you need help to cope with fussy eaters or tantrums?

Feeding your Baby is your sensible and realistic guide to everything a baby needs for a healthy, happy and balanced diet. From breast-feeding and weaning to the needs of the growing child, it has plenty of practical information on every area, with advice on healthy foods, support for mealtime battles and tasty recipes for all ages.

Judy More is the found of the Child Nutrition consultancy. Previously a paediatric dietician for several hospitals and community trusts, she now runs a private consultancy offering nutritional advice to parents and children.

teach
yourself

green parenting
lynoa cattanach

- Do you want advice on natural pregnancy and birth?
- Do you want to be an environmentally aware parent?
- Would you like a happy, healthy and balanced family?

Green Parenting is a practical guide to making informed, ethically aware choices for your family. It covers all elements of domestic life, from children and nappies to travel and toys, offering step-by-step advice and useful suggestions for every level of interest and commitment.

Lynoa Cattanach is a director of BabyGROE, a charity promoting a parent-friendly approach to a greener life through its magazines and website.